Longevity the art of graceful aging

By

Lucy R. Velazquez

Table of content

Introduction

There is now a lot of interest in the relationship between calorie consumption and lifespan. It is still unclear if calorie restriction slows aging or increases longevity.

Increase your intake of nuts; they are nutritional powerhouses high in protein, fibre, antioxidants, and other plant components. Additionally, they are a fantastic source of several vitamins and minerals, including folate, niacin, magnesium, copper, potassium, and vitamins B6 and E.

When it comes to anti-aging methods, turmeric is a fantastic choice. This is because of the presence of curcumin, a powerful bioactive molecule, in this spice.
Curcumin is believed to help preserve brain, heart, and lung function as well as guard against cancer and age-related illnesses

because of its anti-inflammatory and antioxidant characteristics.

Eat a variety of wholesome plant foods. Widespread plant food consumption, including that of fruits, vegetables, nuts, seeds, whole grains, and beans, may lower illness risk and lengthen life.

Additionally, some studies indicate that consuming more meat may raise the risk of certain illnesses and early mortality.

These results may be at least partially explained by the fact that vegetarians and vegans usually value their health more than meat eaters.

Overall, consuming a lot of plant foods may promote longevity and good health. Continue to be active It should not come as a surprise that maintaining a healthy lifestyle will help you live longer

You may see advantages, such as an extra three years of life, with as little as 15 minutes of exercise every day.

Inside this book, you will learn simple strategies and tips to avoid fast aging for life. Sit back, relax, and stay tuned for these life-changing strategies.

Chapter 1

Can You Make Your Life Longer?

Want to know the key to a longer, healthier life? Worms, mice, and even monkeys may now live longer, healthier lives because of scientific advancements. Their research has produced fascinating new hints regarding the biology of aging. Evidence-based guidelines including eating properly, exercising frequently, getting enough sleep, and avoiding poor behaviors are still the greatest ways to increase your chances of living a long and active life. These days, older individuals also tend to be in better health. Healthy habits may keep you active and healthy well into your 60s, 70s, and beyond, according to research. In reality,

a lengthy examination of Seventh-day Adventists, a religious sect with a generally healthy lifestyle, reveals that they frequently maintain their health into old age.

Their average life expectancy is over ten years higher than that of other Americans. Regular exercise, a vegetarian diet, abstaining from alcohol and cigarettes, and keeping a healthy weight are among the Adventists' age-enhancing habits.

Natural aging processes in the body can cause progressive muscle loss, decreased energy, and achy joints. It could be tempting to sit more and move less as a result of these changes. But doing so might increase your danger, death, paralysis, and even. It's crucial to see a doctor identify the physical activities that will support your continued health and mobility. Regular physical exercise is beneficial for elderly persons, including those who are fragile. Over 600 at-risk seniors between the ages of 70 and 89 participated in one NIH-funded research. They were assigned at random to either a moderate exercise program or a control group that did not participate in organized exercise.

The exercise group steadily increased their weekly activity to 150 minutes. This involved vigorous walking, balance, and strength training, and flexibility drills.

"After more than two years, the physical activity group had less impairment, and if they did become impaired, they were incapacitated for a shorter period than those in the comparison group. "Aerobic, strength, balance, and flexibility training along with other forms of exercise are essential for good aging,"

Losing weight is a surefire method to increase your chances of living a longer, healthier life. Obesity, defined as a body mass index (BMI) of 30 or more, reduces active life expectancy and increases the chance of early mortality. Based on your weight and height, your BMI provides an estimate of your body fat. To calculate your BMI, use the NIH BMI calculator.

Animal studies have shown that some dietary modifications, including extremely low-calorie diets, can result in longer, healthier lives. These researches provide indicators of the biological procedures that have an impact on good aging.

However, to date, calorie-restricted diets and other dietary adjustments have had conflicting effects on how long people may live in good health.

Although there is some indirect evidence that dietary changes might increase people's active lifespan, there is still a lot of research to be done in this area. "As of right now, there isn't very strong data concerning calorie restriction and if it may slow down human aging." Researchers are currently looking at possible medications or other strategies that might duplicate the advantages of calorie restriction.

Another approach to live longer, healthier lives is to stop smoking. Smoking is undoubtedly a difficult habit to stop. However, evidence points to health advantages as soon as you stop smoking. Therefore, it is worthwhile to make the effort, You might believe that having healthy genes would help you live longer. Genes, however, only make up a portion of the equation for the majority of us; they only determine less than one-third of your odds of living to be 85 years old living to be 85 years old. Our health behaviors account for the great majority of the difference in how old we live to be. If we live healthy lives, "our genes might get most of us near to the extraordinary age of 90." For those who live longer, such as past the age of 95, the genetic effect is larger. Centenarians and their families gain greater knowledge about the biological, psychological, and social aspects that support good aging.

It appears that no one gene has a significant impact on one's capacity to live into old life Instead, it's the combined impacts of many genes, each with marginal effects on its own, but when coupled correctly, they may have a powerful impact, especially on surviving to the longest ages we have studied.

Be wary of promises of an immediate solution to issues connected to aging. "Anti-aging" strategies like "hormone replacement therapy" can have negative side effects and have no value for healthy aging. The adage, "The older you grow, the sicker you get," used to be true. However, using common sense and good practices like regular exercise, maintaining a healthy weight, avoiding red meat, quitting smoking, and the ability to manage stress can lead to the statement that "the older you are, the healthier you've been.

The secret to good aging is to engage fully in life—mentally, physically, and socially. "Ageing isn't just about kicking back in a rocking chair and watching the years pass you by; older people often have rich life experiences to share with younger generations as well as intellectual and emotional resources.

Stay Healthy

Maintain Your Health by Moving! Exercise can lower your chances of developing age-related illnesses and disabilities.

- Adopt a balanced diet.
- Be mindful of your size and form Health hazards can increase with excess weight, especially around the waist or with muscle loss.
- Quit smoking and using tobacco.
- Maintain mental activity.
- Take care of yourself. Obtain adequate rest.

- Keep in contact with your loved ones and friends. Also, surround yourself with like-minded individuals.
- .Attend routine medical checks.
- If you consume alcohol, do it only seldom.

When we consider health and longevity, we frequently picture medical professionals caring for patients. And yet, throughout human evolution and history, human health has improved more because we tend not to get sick rather than because of what happens to us when we do. Because of safer environments

 (Sanitation and clean water), improved diet, and the innate healing and self-regulatory abilities of the human body, we also tend not to get sick.

In other words, the physical and social environment, human behavior, and heredity, together with medical treatment to a lesser extent, are the main determinants of human health in both developed and developing countries are our genetics, physical and social environments, human behavior, and, to a lesser extent, medical care.

The majority of the world's population is seeing an increase in life expectancy; the outliers are primarily the result of war, diseases, and societal upheaval. Instead of treating the sick after they become ill, medical treatment is still mainly responsible for the increases in life expectancy in public health and preventative measures (some of which are supplied through medical care).

It is remarkable how little medical advancements over the entire 20th century increased life expectancy.

Life expectancy climbed by 8.8 years between 1950 and 2000 (years that corresponded with the expansion in medical technology in the United States),
but by 20.9 years from 1900 to 1950, a period when medicine frequently had little to offer in the way of significant treatments. Before the development of a cure or vaccine for these diseases, the death rates for the infectious diseases that were the main causes of death throughout this period significantly decreased.

More years have been added to human life expectancy as a result of rising quality of living and related advancements in housing, sanitation, and nutrition than all elements of medical treatment put together.

The capacity of improvements in the standard or use of medical treatment to lower American death rates is rather constrained. Given that we spend 17.8% of our gross domestic product (GDP) on healthcare, this is fairly remarkable. This is almost double what other industrialized nations spend on average. However, the US has a lower life expectancy than comparable nations.

In the 20th century, improved medical treatment was responsible for around five of the thirty years of enhanced life expectancy. As technology improves and is better equipped to meet the healthcare demands of our aging population, the relative contribution of medical care to life expectancy increased in the late half of the 20th century. This trend is expected to continue.

The advantages of medical treatment also have expenses, both monetary and physical. Health suffers as a result of medical mistakes, incorrect diagnoses, hospital-acquired infections, negative side effects, drug addiction, etc.

Approximately 2-4 percent of all deaths in the US, or 44,000–98,00 deaths each year, may be directly attributable to medical mistakes.

The amount, according to the Centers for Disease Control and Prevention (CDC), deficits in the healthcare system account for around 10% of all deaths. According to estimates, 142,000 persons worldwide passed away in 2013 as a result of negative medical treatment outcomes, up from 94,000 in 1990. You might think of heart disease, stroke, cancer, infections, accidents, and other conditions as the causes of mortality and incapacity. However, a distinct image materializes upon examination of the underlying causes of these particular diseases. Using the most accurate estimates, the influence of different domains on early fatalities in the United States broadly follows the distribution as follows:

- genetic predisposition; 30%
- Social environment: 15%
- Environmental exposures: 5%
- Attitude and way of life: 40%
- Health care: 10%

The interactions between each of these areas, however, are more significant than the ratios. Environmental exposures or behavioral tendencies may influence the expression of a gene. Our social circumstances have an impact on the type and results of behavioral decisions. Both our social surroundings and our genetic predispositions influence the healthcare we require and receive.

Our social circumstances have an impact on the type and results of behavioral decisions. Both our social surroundings and our genetic predispositions influence the healthcare we require and receive.

How well do our health investments, in light of this viewpoint, represent the real determinants of health?

About 95% of the billions of dollars that the US spends on health as a country goes into direct medical care, with just 5% going towards population-wide strategies for health improvement.

However, behavior patterns that may be changed by preventative measures are responsible for around 40% of fatalities. The leading causes of mortality in developed nations include smoking, inactivity, a poor diet, and heavy alcohol use.

In actuality, it appears that a significantly lower share of avoidable death in the United States may be prevented by improved access to or the caliber of medical treatment, probably 10-15 percent. Therefore, one can question a financial reality that prioritizes medical treatment so much at the expense of prevention. Of course, longevity does not represent a person's overall health. The typical individual now lives with a handicap for a longer period as a result of longer lifespans. Major depressive illness, anxiety disorder, low back and neck pain, and other musculoskeletal problems were the main causes of years lived with disability in the US.

Sometimes, medical intervention can significantly enhance a person's ability to manage certain conditions. One example is the remarkable increase in quality of life that can come after a successful hip replacement. The main avenues for enhancing the quality of life and functioning, however, once more point to altering food, boosting physical activity, abstaining from cigarette use and excessive alcohol use, as well as controlling stress. Additionally, in underdeveloped nations, access to clean water, better diet, and immunizations continue to be important health-related factors.

Not that medical treatment is unimportant—far from it. In actuality, the careful use of medical science from drugs to surgery—saves or at least improves countless lives. Instead, we overestimate the influence of healthcare on human health, and as a result, many individuals experience abuse or overtreatment in addition to a lack of access to efficient, evidence-based healthcare.

Understanding the cause of any ailment might make treating it simpler. A person's genetic makeup, lifestyle choices (like smoking), exposure to harmful chemicals (like asbestos), and other factors can all contribute to health issues. When dealing with several health issues, one disease or its treatment may trigger another.

After a protracted period of ambiguity, maybe including several tests and investigations or being sent to a variety of medical specialists, the cause of a condition may finally be discovered. Sometimes people develop ailments for which they have no apparent cause. In the absence of a medical explanation, a person may develop their theories, such as that it was just "poor luck."

Chapter 2
What is Exercise Science?

We all know that exercise is important in our daily lives, but we may not know why or what exercise can do for us. It's important to remember that we have evolved from nomadic ancestors who spent all their time moving around in search of food and shelter, traveling large distances daily. Our bodies are designed and have evolved to be regularly active.

Exercise Science is a discipline that studies movement and the associated functional responses and adaptations.

The goal of exercise science is to facilitate an understanding of the links between fitness, exercise, diet, and health. Ultimately, the discipline provides a scientific approach to studying how exercise and the human body interact to understand the physiology of exercise as well as its benefits and results. Exercise Science encompasses a wide variety of disciplines and the study of these disciplines is integrated into the academic preparation of exercise science professionals.

Disciplines include areas such as biomechanics, sports nutrition, sport and exercise psychology, motor control and development, and exercise physiology. In addition, the coursework includes evaluating health behaviors and risk factors, conducting fitness assessments, writing appropriate exercise prescriptions, and promoting positive health habits and lifestyle behaviors.

Exercise science professionals are part of a multidisciplinary team whose work ranges from helping people recover from the unhealthy effects of a sedentary lifestyle to assisting athletes to perform at their maximum capability.

You will find exercise science professionals in a variety of disciplines, such as:

- College Sport Teams

- Human and Athletic Performance Centers

- Fitness and Wellness Centers

- Hospital Fitness and Rehabilitation Centers

- University and industry research laboratories

- Weight control programs

Why exercise?

Exercise is a powerful medicine. Exercise is an important part of a healthy lifestyle. Exercise prevents health problems, builds strength, boosts energy, and can help you reduce stress. It can also help you maintain a healthy body weight and curb your appetite.

Exercise can:

- Reduce your risk of heart disease, high blood pressure, osteoporosis, diabetes, and obesity.

- Reduce your risk of breast, colorectal, and uterine cancer.

- Keep your bones, muscles, joints, tendons, and ligaments flexible, which makes it easier to move around and decreases your chance of falling.

- Reduce some of the effects of aging, especially the discomfort of osteoarthritis.

- Contribute to mental well-being and help treat depression.

- Help relieve stress, depression, and anxiety.

- Increase energy and endurance.

- Improved sleep helps you maintain a normal weight by increasing your metabolism (the rate at which you burn calories).

- Help with your balance, so you're less likely to fall and break bones.

How much exercise?

You don't have to become an elite athlete to improve your longevity. Regular, moderate activities, such as brisk walking, have been associated with increasing life expectancy by several years. For example, 150 minutes of exercise or more each week increased life expectancy by about 7 years over those who didn't do regular moderate exercise. This benefit was seen regardless of weight, age, sex, and health conditions.

If you haven't been active or are thinking of increasing your activity, be sure to talk with your doctor. Based on your current health, your doctor may have recommendations for the type of activity and how much to get you started.

As you get older, you may be a bit afraid of exercise. Maybe you think you might hurt yourself or that you have to join a gym. Or you may not be sure what exercises you should do.

Potential Careers in Exercise Science

Fitness Facilities

Graduates from the Exercise Science programs have the academic preparation to work in a variety of fitness settings. Commercial fitness facilities are those that are operated on a for-profit basis. Examples of commercial fitness facilities include Gold's Gym, Anytime Fitness, 24 Hour Fitness, or CrossFit boxes. Corporate fitness facilities are owned by a business but typically operated by an outside agency. For instance, many federal government offices have a corporate fitness facility. An example of a corporate fitness company is Corporate Fitness Works. Hospital-based fitness facilities may either be on a hospital campus or at a satellite location. They are also known as medical fitness facilities and often have members who have medically controlled conditions. Locally, an example is the Sentara RMH Wellness Center. Community fitness facilities are operated on a not-for-profit basis. Examples of this type of facility include YMCAs or parks and recreation departments.

Medical Opportunities

There are many possibilities for students who are interested in employment in health care. Oftentimes, this type of employment will require at least two more years of education after the completion of a bachelor's degree, depending on your interests. The following opportunities are examples, but not an inclusive list:

- Physical Therapy
- Physical Therapy Assistant
- Rehabilitation Technician
- Occupational Therapy
- Recreational Therapy
- Physician Assistant
- Surgical Technician

Additional Opportunities exercise science is a broad curriculum, there are many ways a person might use their degree after graduation. The Kinesiology faculty, Kinesiology academic adviser, and Career and Academic Planning Office are available to talk about your interests and potential career paths. The following opportunities are examples, but not an inclusive list:

- Personal Trainer

- Exercise Physiologist

- Sports Physiologist

- Cardiac Rehabilitation

- Nutrition and Exercise Specialist

- Health Care Specialist

- Basic and Applied Sciences

- Graduate program study

Regular physical activity is one of the most important things you can do for your health. Being physically active can improve your brain health, help manage your weight, reduce the risk of disease, strengthen your bones and muscles, and improve your ability to do everyday activities.

How much exercise do I need?

A good goal is to exercise five times a week for at least 30 minutes each time. However, most people need to start gradually. Start by exercising 2 or 3 times a week for 20 minutes at a time. Once you feel comfortable, slowly increase the amount of time and the number of days a week that you exercise.

How hard do I have to exercise to gain health benefits?

Even small amounts of exercise are better than none at all. Start with an activity you enjoy and can do comfortably. Learn to take your pulse and calculate your target heart rate (about 80% of your "maximum heart rate"). As you become used to exercising, try to exercise within your target heart rate zone so that you get the most benefit. However, discuss this with your doctor before beginning. Exercising at 80% of your target heart rate may not be appropriate for everyone. This is especially true if you have certain health conditions or are taking medications.

To take your pulse, gently rest two fingers on the side of your neck, about halfway between your ear and your chin. Count the beats for 10 seconds. Multiply this number by 6 to get the number of beats per minute. For example, if you are sitting still and counting 12 beats over 10 seconds, multiply 12 by 6 to get 72 beats per minute.

To figure out your target heart rate, subtract your age (in years) from 220. This is your maximum heart rate. To calculate your target heart rate, multiply that number by 0.80.

For example, if you are 40 years of age, subtract 40 from 220, which gives you a maximum heart rate of 180 (220 minus 40 = 180). Then multiply this number by 0.80, which gives 144 (180 x 0.80 =144). Your target heart rate would be 144 beats per minute.

Track your progress.

Keep a record of your workouts to track your progress. Write down how long you exercised and what you did. Free websites are available to track your progress, as well as apps for smartphones (one app: MyFitnessPal).

Find an exercise partner.

Working out with a friend is more fun than working out alone. An exercise buddy can keep you motivated when you don't feel like exercising. You will be much less likely to cancel exercise if you know someone is counting on you to be there. And when you reach your exercise goals, you'll have someone to celebrate with.

Things to consider

To avoid injuring yourself during exercise, don't try to do too much too soon. Start with an activity that is fairly easy for you, such as walking. Do it for a few minutes a day, several times a day. Slowly increase the amount of time and the intensity of the activity. For example, increase your walking time and speed over several weeks.

Trying to push yourself too hard, in the beginning, could cause muscle strain or sprain. When this happens, you'll have to wait for the injury to heal before continuing your exercise program. This can sidetrack your health goals.

When to see a doctor

Pay attention to your body. Stop exercising if you feel very out of breath, dizzy, faint, nauseous, or if you feel pain. Talk with your family doctor if you have questions or think you have injured yourself seriously.

Questions to ask your doctor

- Am I healthy enough to begin an exercise program?

- Are there any exercises I should avoid?

- Do I have any health conditions that would affect my ability to exercise?

- Am I taking any medication that would interfere with exercise?

Can anyone exercise?

Everyone can benefit from physical activity. For most people, it is possible to begin exercising on their own at a slow pace. If you have never exercised before, start with 10 minutes of light exercise. A brisk walk every day is a good first exercise. Slowly increase how hard you exercise and for how long.

Talk to your doctor before starting an exercise program. This is especially important if your doctor is already monitoring you for a health problem, such as heart disease or osteoarthritis. You should try to exercise even if you have a physical disability that limits movement. Your doctor can help you find other exercises to improve your overall health.

We have all heard it many times before regular exercise is good for you, and it can help you lose weight. But if you are like many Americans, you are busy, you have a sedentary job, and you haven't yet changed your exercise habits. The good news is that it's never too late to start. You can start slowly and find ways to fit more physical activity into your life. To get the most benefit, you should try to get the recommended amount of exercise for your age. If you can do it, the payoff is that you will feel better, help prevent or control many diseases, and likely even live longer.

What are the health benefits of exercise?

Regular exercise and physical activity may:

Help you control your weight. Along with diet, exercise plays an important role in controlling your weight and preventing obesity. To maintain your weight, the calories you eat and drink must equal the energy you burn. To lose weight, you must use more calories than you eat and drink. Exercise improves both the strength and the efficiency of your cardiovascular system to get oxygen and nutrients to your muscles. When your cardiovascular system works better, everything seems easier, and you have more energy for the fun stuff in life. The more you exercise, the more calories you burn. In addition, the more muscle you develop, the higher your metabolic rate becomes, so you burn more calories even when you're not exercising. The result? You may lose weight and look better physically, which will boost your self-esteem.

Reduce your risk of heart disease. Exercise strengthens your heart and improves your circulation. The increased blood flow raises the oxygen levels in your body. This helps lower your risk of heart diseases such as high cholesterol, coronary artery disease, and heart attack. Regular exercise can also lower your blood pressure and triglyceride levels. Exercise reduces LDL cholesterol (the type that clogs your arteries), increases HDL (the good cholesterol), and reduces blood pressure, so it lowers the stress on your heart. Added to this, it also strengthens your heart muscle. Combined with a healthy diet, exercise lowers the risk of developing coronary heart disease.

Help your body manage blood sugar and insulin levels. Exercise can lower your blood sugar level and help your insulin work well. This can cut down on your risk for metabolic syndrome and type 2 diabetes. And if you already have one of those diseases, exercise can help you manage it.

Help you quit smoking. Exercise may make it easier to quit_smoking by reducing your cravings and withdrawal symptoms. It can also help limit the weight you might gain when you stop smoking.

Improve your mental health and mood. During exercise, your body releases chemicals that can improve your mood and make you feel more relaxed. This can help you deal with stress and reduce your risk of depression.

Physical activity stimulates the release of endorphins, which make you feel better and more relaxed. These, in turn, improve your mood and lower your stress levels.

Help keep your thinking, learning, and judgment skills sharp as you age. Exercise stimulates your body to release proteins and other chemicals that improve the structure and function of your brain.

Strengthen your bones and muscles. Regular exercise can help kids and teens build strong bones. Later in life, it can also slow the loss of bone density that comes with age. Doing muscle-strengthening activities can help you increase or maintain your muscle mass and strength.

Reduce your risk of some cancers, including colon, breast, uterine, and lung

Reduce your risk of falling. For older adults, research shows that doing balance and muscle-strengthening activities in addition to moderate-intensity aerobic activity can help reduce your risk of falling.

Improve your sleep. Exercise can help you fall asleep faster and stay asleep longer. Physical activity makes you more tired, so you're more ready to sleep. Good-quality sleep helps improve overall wellness and can reduce stress.

Improve your sexual health. Regular exercise may lower the risk of erectile dysfunction (ED) in men. For those who already have ED, exercise may help improve their sexual function. In women, exercise may increase sexual arousal.

Increase your chances of living longer. Studies show that physical activity can reduce your risk of dying early from the leading causes of death, like heart disease and some cancers.

How can I make exercise a part of my routine?

Make everyday activities more active. Even small changes can help. You can take the stairs instead of the elevator. Walk down the hall to a coworker's office instead of sending an email. Wash the car yourself. Park further away from your destination.

Be active with friends and family. Having a workout partner may make you more likely to enjoy exercise. You can also plan social activities that involve exercise. You might also consider joining an exercise group or class, such as a dance class, hiking club, or volleyball team.

Keep track of your progress. Keeping a log of your activity or using a fitness tracker may help you set goals and stay motivated.

Make exercise more fun. Try listening to music or watching TV while you exercise. Also, mix things up a little bit; if you stick with just one type of exercise, you might get bored. Try doing a combination of activities.

Find activities that you can do even when the weather is bad. You can walk in a mall, climb stairs, or work out in a gym even if the weather stops you from exercising outside.

Health Benefits of Exercise That May Surprise You

You have heard it for years—the health benefits of exercise can't be denied.

Despite any dismay you feel towards sweating, research indicates regular sweat sessions are good for both your physical and mental health.

Other than looking good and feeling strong, the list of benefits of regular exercise is quite long. Some of the perks may even surprise you, like delayed aging and reduce bodily inflammation.

If you're looking for a reason to keep up your workout routine into the fall and holiday season, your list of exercise incentives is here.

Here are some surprising health benefits of exercise to get you excited to sweat—even if it's just a little bit.

Weekly exercise improves your health in a variety of ways.

The Department of Health and Human Services recommends adults mix up routines between strength training and aerobic activity for the best results.

To achieve maximum health benefits, fitting in 150 minutes of weekly aerobic activity should be the minimum amount you strive for. Or 75 minutes of vigorous activity a week. Pair that with strength training twice a week, and you'll be well on your way to better health.

Make it feel more doable by setting a goal of 30 minutes of physical activity daily. That can even be split into two 15-minute sessions if you can't carve out a full half-hour. The important thing is to make it a regular part of your healthy lifestyle choices.

Now, here's a look at the health benefits of exercise:

1. May Delay Signs of aging

Your skin—the body's largest organ—can be negatively impacted by oxidative stress inside the body. Oxidative stress risk factors include obesity, alcohol consumption, and poor diets, all of which can damage cell structures. Luckily, regular, moderate exercise is known to increase natural antioxidants to protect your body's cells. Exercise also promotes blood flow, which can give you a post-workout glow as well as delay the appearance of aging skin like wrinkles. Hello, natural facelift!

2. minimizes bodily inflammation

If you struggle with inflammatory diseases, like arthritis, exercise can help you lubricate your joints and feel better overall. Regular exercise is proven to reduce chronic inflammation, according to research. That's because the body is forced to adapt to exercise challenges. Even a single moderate exercise session can act as an anti-inflammatory for issues like fibromyalgia, according to a University of California San Diego School of Medicine study.

3. **helps with emotional processing**

If you've been neglecting your self-care, it's time to invest in yourself. During stressful times, exercise can be an excellent form of self-care, especially when you're in high-pressure environments. Heading out for a walk in nature, for example, is a great way to exercise and also allows space away from life obligations to simply process emotions. Research proves that spending at least 120 minutes a week in nature is good for your overall well-being. Those benefits double when you spend it walking or exercising, too!

4. Gives you more energy.

Do you think exercise will make you feel even more exhausted? It's unlikely, studies show. If you usually turn to soda or another energy booster during the day, opting for exercise can be a better choice for sustained energy. Consistent exercise is shown to reduce fatigue and improve energy levels overall. Even low-intensity exercise like walking has been shown to reduce fatigue symptoms by up to 65 percent!

5. Improves Learning

Looking for a brain boost? Start exercising. Activities that require extreme concentration—like dance or tennis—challenge the mind and coordination. This causes growth factor brain chemicals to grow and expand to help us learn. Consistent exercise can also improve concentration and attention.

6. **gives mental clarity**

Between remote work, family obligations, professional commitments, and more, life can feel like a never-ending to-do list. If you tend to be in problem-solving mode most of the day, exercise can give you an escape for the moment. When you move your body, you're focusing on just moving your body and getting into the present moment. Doing so reduces cortisol levels, offers some mental clarity that doesn't involve "what's next?" and allows you to settle into the present.

7. **offers a natural, healthy**

If you've heard about "runner's high," then you likely know exercise is proven to offer a huge mental boost. Even if you don't love running, other activities like hot yoga or power walking offer an endorphin release that provides a euphoric feeling. Those happy hormones can keep you feeling upbeat and peppy for the rest of the day, giving a natural, healthy "high" to those who invest in exercise time.

8. lifts the spirit

Sometimes you need a boost that can't be found by just binge-watching your favorite shows. Exercise is a perfect way to build stress relief into the day as an opportunity to refresh your outlook and recharge mentally. Not only does the body physically benefit from exercise—whether it's walking or kickboxing—but you'll see overall mental and emotional health benefits, too.

9. Weight training equals calories burned during rest.

Enjoy weight training? Other than feeling like a superhuman who can lift heavy stuff, the benefit of this exercise is clear: consistent weight training will help you burn more calories even during a restful state. The more calories burned during a workout, the more you burn after the workout as well!

10. Exercise Benefits the Body Within Weeks

If you've been a couch potato for the last 5 years, remember that you won't lose weight overnight. You also won't be able to run a marathon the first day you step into your workout routine. As you exercise regularly, you gain more fitness benefits. Experts say within six to eight weeks you'll notice health benefits—like it's easier to climb that flight of stairs than before.

11. Cardiovascular disease reduces significantly

When conditions like heart disease run in your family, it's essential to be continuously mindful of ways to stay healthy. Exercise and diet are the top two ways to keep your heart health in check, especially if you have a family history of heart conditions. One study found that those who do the most physical activity can lower their cardiovascular risk by 60 percent. Additionally, consistent exercise routines after age 60 can prevent stroke and heart disease.

12. Safely reduces blood pressure

A new study from the University of New South Wales found a simple way to lower pressure—without meds—isometric resistance training (IRT). IRT is a type of strength training where the muscles produce force but do not length, — like holding the plank position. Exercise physiologists found IRT to be safe for those with high blood pressure and quite effective at lower A billion people globally have high blood pressure. High blood pressure increases the risk of stroke or heart attack and exercise is a recommended management technique for those with the condition.

13. Decreases PMS

For women who suffer from extreme irritation or bloating before their menstrual cycles, surprisingly, exercise can minimize both conditions. One New Zealand survey of 2,000 women found that those who worked out, rested, and journaled about their symptoms did better than those who took vitamins or used other DIY advice.

14. Catch more quality ZZZs.

Insomnia and sleep issues not only impact your energy but also your quality of life. If you opt to regularly commit to an exercise routine, you're more likely to improve your sleep quality. Moderate aerobic exercise increases slow-wave sleep, also known as deep sleep—an essential part of the sleep cycle that lets the body's cells rejuvenate.

15. Specific breathing techniques are a workout.

If the thought of getting sweaty grosses you out, start with a simple yet effective exercise: strength training for breathing muscles. Not only does it improve blood pressure as well as aerobic exercise, but it is also shown to reduce inflammation markers. The breathing exercise inspiratory muscle Strength training is shown to reduce blood pressure within weeks,

It's never too late to be active.

No matter how old you are, it's never too late to start benefiting from exercise. The immediate effects are noticeable and worth it, even for light exercise activities like yoga or tai chi. Loose muscles, lower blood pressure, and feeling a sense of accomplishment are instant gratifications you'll get from exercise, no matter how old you are or how long it's been since your last sweat session.

Find your reason to like exercise.

You don't have to love exercise. But finding an exercise activity you *like* enough to do consistently can help you reap the above health benefits.

Try a fun activity to do alone, with friends, or in a group to get the most out of your exercise routines. Anything from tennis to running groups or even power walking daily counts towards your exercise goals!

A few more interesting facts about exercise:

Chewing gum makes you walk harder. Gum chewing while walking can increase your energy expenditure and walking distance if you're middle-aged, according to one study published in July 2021 in the Journal of Exercise Science & Fitness.

Chocolate may improve fat burn in women—yes, you read that right. Brigham and Women's Hospital published a study that found postmenopausal women who eat a concentrated amount of milk chocolate during a specific time frame in the morning may help the body burn fat along with decreasing blood sugar levels. The small study found that eating 100 grams of milk chocolate within an hour of waking could reduce hunger and the desire for sweets. Additionally, for early morning workouts, an evening chocolate treat helped with next-day exercise metabolism.

There you have it—even more reasons than ever to keep your health in check and exercise scheduled on the calendar. As always, consult your physician before starting any fitness routine, especially if you have pre-existing conditions or medications that may impact your workouts or health.

Wondering where to start?

There's a place to start for everyone, regardless of age or current fitness level.

First, think about safety. Walking and other low-level exercises are generally safe for most people. But check with your doctor before starting or making changes to an exercise routine if you have a history of heart disease or any other medical condition that might impact your exercise tolerance.

Start small. You'll be more successful if you set the bar low. For example, start with a simple routine of walking 10 to 20 minutes three times per week. Every week or two, add five minutes per walk until you reach a goal of 30 minutes. Then, every week or two, add a day until you reach at least 150 minutes per week. Over time, you can try to increase the intensity. Remember, small goals are more achievable, and these little victories will continue to fuel your motivation.

Don't be afraid of exercise or the gym. Any movement is good and is a step in the right direction. The gym intimidates many folks—

perhaps you're overweight or inexperienced and worry that others might stare at you or judge you. Everyone was new to exercise at one point in time. Focus on your purpose and avoid wasting energy on things that do not matter.

Plan. To maximize your success in adopting a long-term lifestyle change, plan. Look at your calendar ahead of time every week and commit to when you will exercise that week. Think of your opportunity to exercise as an appointment, rather than "I'll get to it if I have time."

Expect to lose some battles. Keep in mind that, realistically, most people will get derailed at some point as they work on a behavioral change. Do not let this crush your motivation. Instead, identify obstacles that may have interfered, strategize a solution moving forward, and try again.

Can exercise extend your life?

Does exercise help you live longer?

Multiple studies have shown that regular weekly exercise increases your lifespan. Others have shown that a lack of exercise can shorten your life. For example, research found that for Americans between the ages of 40 and 70, 10% of deaths can be attributed to not exercising enough. A separate analysis found that the risk of death for physically active individuals is 20 to 35% lower than for someone who doesn't exercise. Two studies, which followed more than 10,000 adults over several decades, reached a similar conclusion: certain types and amounts of exercise can reduce one's risk of prematurely dying by up to 70%.

A comprehensive review found that those who partake in regular physical activity can increase their life expectancy by 2 to 4 years, and this was a conservative estimate. Researchers predicted it could be even greater because of exercise's ability to decrease major risk factors attributed to mortality. Regular exercise in combination with four other healthy lifestyle factors, including not smoking, maintaining a healthy weight, eating a healthy diet, and drinking alcohol in moderation, can prolong a 50-year-old female's life by 14 years and extend a male's life by 12.2 years.

How does exercise increase your life expectancy?

It helps prevent excessive weight gain. Exercise burns calories and increases muscle mass, helping with weight loss and maintenance. More muscle increases your metabolism, the rate at which your body burns calories, and when paired with consuming fewer calories, it can help create a deficit for weight loss. A study by a subsidiary of the National Institutes of Health found that extreme obesity can shorten a lifespan by up to 14 years.

It helps prevent and manage health conditions. There are numerous conditions that physical activity can help with, **including:**

- Life-expectancy;

- Stroke;

- Metabolic syndrome;

- High blood pressure;

- Type 2 diabetes

- Depression;

- Anxiety;

- There are many types of cancer.

- Arthritis.

It makes you happier and more confident. Exercise increases endorphins, making you feel cheerier, calmer, and more optimistic. Physical activity can also boost your confidence, causing you to feel better about yourself. Optimistic people have been shown to have a longer life span and an increased chance of living past 85.

It increases your energy. Physical activity adds muscle, improves your endurance, circulates oxygen and nutrients throughout the body, and keeps your cardiovascular system in tip-top shape. You'll feel more energized to tackle the day's to-do list, and you can reduce your risk of heart disease.

It helps you sleep better. Exercise helps with falling asleep faster and improves the quality of your sleep. Not getting enough sleep is another factor linked to premature death, so it's important to get the recommended 7 to 8 hours each night.

It acts as an anti-inflammatory.

Exercise provides the body with an anti-inflammatory effect. Inflammation increases the risk of disease, death, and loss of physical function.

It improves digestion. Exercise can positively change your gut microbial composition, which improves your overall health and helps prevent disease.

It encourages socialization. Whether you do it with friends or family, going for a walk or hike, joining a recreational team, or training for a race together is a great way to meet with friends and work up a sweat at the same time. Research shows that people with more friends can outlive those with fewer friends by 22%.

Exercise provides a remarkable variety of health benefits, which range from strengthening bones to positive effects on mood and helping to prevent chronic illnesses such as diabetes and heart disease. Research dating back to the late 1980s has consistently shown that aerobic fitness may help extend lives. Yet a few studies on athletes examining whether habitual vigorous exercise might harm the heart made some experts wonder how hard people ought to push when exercising.

Want to live longer? Get moving.

We all know that exercise can help you get fit, reduce weight, improve balance, and lower your risk for many diseases, such as heart disease. However numerous studies have shown that exercise can help you live longer.

This seems logical. After all, if exercise reduces your chance of getting heart disease or cancer, then you've reduced your risk of dying from these diseases. However, the longevity benefit is not just a result of reducing your risk of chronic disease. There are actual cellular changes associated with regular exercise that keep you younger.

Longevity; the art of graceful aging

Researchers at Brigham Young University who studied the DNA of nearly 6,000 adults found that the telomeres, the end caps on chromosomes that shorten with age, were longer in people who were active compared to those who were sedentary. This correlated to a 9-year difference in cell aging between those who were active and those who were inactive.

Another study compared the heart, lungs, and muscles of active 70-year-olds, inactive 70-year-olds, and active 40-year-olds. They found that the active older men and women had comparable heart and lung capacity and muscle strength to those who were 30 years younger.

Exercise results in other physiological changes that can help slow the aging process: as we see above.

- It is anti-inflammatory. Inflammation of muscles and other tissues in the body is associated with aging. Exercise can lessen this effect.

- Boost mood

- Improve sleep

- Improve cognitive function and reduce memory loss.

- Improved immune system

- Improved digestive function

It's never too late to start exercising.

Even if you have been sedentary for many years, it's not too late to reap the benefits of exercise. Studies have found that people who are overweight or who have been inactive for years can increase their life expectancy by adding moderate physical activity to their routine.

The key isn't how or where you get active; it's just to start moving.

Healthy adults should aim for 150 minutes of activity that gets your heart going and your blood pumping every week. Sure, you can do that in exercise classes. But you can also get it by briskly walking. It's also important to do movements that work all your major muscles at least twice a week. Also, try to do flexibility exercises 2 or 3 days a week to help with your range of motion.

While 150 minutes may sound like a lot, you don't have to do it in big chunks. You can take a 10-minute walk around the block or spend 10 minutes sweeping the porch. It all adds up.

If you're feeling energetic, you'll get even more health benefits if you work up to 300 minutes or more of exercise a week.

But a simple goal is to try to get 30 minutes of moderate-intensity exercise on most days. You may be able to do that some weeks and not others. Remember, it's a goal and not a rule. Do what works for you.

Tips to begin exercising

Talk to your doctor. Make sure you get a physical before starting a new workout program. Let your practitioner know you're starting a new routine and discuss any concerns you may have. If you have any medical conditions, they can make recommendations on the best exercises or recommend you meet with an exercise physiologist.

Set goals. These don't need to be major goals. They can be as simple as walking five to ten extra minutes in the coming week.

Start small and slow.

Make sure to **warm up and cool down**. You'll prevent injuries and improve flexibility.

Stay hydrated.

If starting a new workout routine feels overwhelming, **seek help from a certified fitness professional**, who can help you create goals and a safe and effective workout regimen.

Exercise ideas for longevity

The great news about exercising for longevity is that no one type of physical activity is better than another. This finding means there are many activities to choose from, making reaching your weekly exercise goal much more attainable. Here are some ideas to get you started.

Endurance and aerobic activities:

- Brisk walking;
- Cycling;
- Jogging;

- Swimming;

- Dancing;

- Rock climbing;

- Jumping rope;

- Jumping on a trampoline

- Climbing hills or stairs;

- Recreational sports, such as basketball, tennis, football, or soccer.

Functional exercise ideas:

- Mowing the lawn

- Housework;

- Yardwork;

- Walking to and from the grocery store rather than driving

- Being active with your children

Strength training ideas:

- Bodyweight exercises;

- Dumbbells routines;

- Using weight machines;

- Working out with resistance bands

How much is too much?

There is a point of diminishing returns when it comes to exercising. The same study that found life expectancy benefits with exercising 2.6 to 4.5 hours weekly also found the group who worked out for 10 or more hours per week, or 90 minutes each day, saw a third fewer mortality benefits compared to the group who exercised less each day. Similarly, the study that examined daily steps found that people who took more than 10,000 steps per day didn't receive additional life expectancy benefits compared to the group who took 7,000 steps each day.

Experts recommend at least 150 minutes of moderate aerobic activity, which includes things such as brisk walking, or 75 minutes of vigorous aerobic activity weekly, including things such as jogging, running, or plyometric. For even more health benefits and to help with weight loss, guidelines suggest at least 300 minutes a week. In addition to aerobic activity, it's important to strength-train each major muscle group at least twice a week.

A systematic review that contributed to Canada's physical activity guidelines found that regular exercise is an effective strategy for helping prevent premature mortality, heart disease, stroke, hypertension, colon and breast cancer, and type 2 diabetes.

Here is the amount of exercise needed to increase your longevity:

A comprehensive analysis of 15 studies examining almost 50,000 people found that adults 60 and older who took between 6,000 and 8,000 steps per day decreased the risk of premature death. Those under 60 should get between 8,000 and 10,000 steps each day to reduce their risk.

Separate research found that 7,000 steps each day reduced premature death in the middle-aged demographic by 50 to 70%.

Exercising between 2.6 and 4.5 hours weekly, which equates to 30 to 45 minutes daily, can increase your lifespan. A study that followed thousands of participants over decades found that those who got 30 to 45 minutes of daily exercise were around 40% less likely to have died than less active study participants.

A separate study found that regular exercise can add 3 to 5 years to one's lifespan.

The bottom line: Depending on your age, aim for between 6,000 and 10,000 steps daily or 30 to 45 minutes of daily exercise. If these numbers seem overwhelming, don't be discouraged. You don't need to jump from

1,000 steps a day to 7,000 overnight. Start small and work towards increasing your exercise minutes each week. Multiple studies have shown that even small amounts of exercise are better than no exercise.

Chapter 3

How to find the right eating pattern for you

For example, each week, try eating several types of vegetables, including dark green, red, and orange, starchy ones, legumes, and others. Switch up the protein foods you eat, too—for example, consider fish, black beans, and peanut butter, not just lean meats and poultry. Try to eat and drink the right amounts for you.

How to build a

Healthy Eating Pattern

There are many different ways to eat healthy. You can eat healthy in a way that works for you and your family. Healthy eating can fit all tastes and traditions—and can be affordable, too.

The key is to build a healthy eating pattern, which means choosing a variety of nutritious foods in the right amounts for you and making these choices part of your everyday routine.

Follow these tips, based on the

2015–2020 Dietary Guidelines for Americans—for Making Choices

that can help you reach or keep a healthy body weight, get the nutrients you need, and lower your risk of health problems like heart disease, type 2 diabetes, and some types of cancer.

Get a variety of nutritious foods and beverages.

Eating a variety of foods and beverages is important. It helps you get the range of nutrients you need to be healthy.

- Eat a mix of foods across all food groups.

Choose foods and beverages from all food groups—vegetables, fruits, grains, dairy, and proteins—not just one or two of them.

Vegetables

Fruits, especially whole fruits

Grains, especially whole grains

Fat-free and low-fat dairy, including milk, yogurt, cheese, and fortified soy beverages

Protein foods, like seafood, lean meats and poultry, eggs, legumes (beans and peas), nuts, seeds, and soy products

- Eat a mix of foods within each food group.

For example, each week, try eating several types of vegetables, including dark green, red, and orange, starchy ones, legumes, and others. Switch up the protein foods you eat, too—for example, consider fish, black beans, and peanut butter, not just lean meats and poultry.

Limit foods and beverages high in saturated fats, added sugars, and sodium.

Less than 10% of calories each day come from saturated fats.

Foods higher in saturated fats include butter, cheese, whole milk, meats higher in fat (like beef ribs, sausage, and some processed meats), poultry skin, and tropical oils like coconut and palm oil. Instead, go for foods with unsaturated fats, like seafood, avocados, most nuts, and canola or olive oil.

Less than 10% of calories each day come from added sugars.

Added sugars are syrups or other sweeteners with calories that are added to foods and drinks when they're being made or prepared. Stick mostly to foods and drinks with naturally occurring sugars—like those in unflavored milk and fruits—or no sugar at all. Choose water instead of sugary drinks, and limit sweet treats like cake, cookies, brownies, and candy.

Less than 2,300 milligrams of sodium each day for adults and children ages 14 and up (less for younger children)

Sodium comes from table salt, but most of the sodium we eat comes from foods that are packaged or served in restaurants. When buying foods in the store, check the Nutrition Facts label and choose the option with the lowest amount of sodium. To cut down on sodium, cook more at home or ask not to have salt added to your meal when eating out.

Small changes equal big benefits.

Small shifts in your daily eating habits can improve your health over the long run. For example, try swapping out white bread for whole-wheat bread and reaching for a handful of nuts instead of potato chips.

Stick with it.

A lifetime of healthy eating can help prevent health problems like obesity, heart disease, type 2 diabetes, and some types of cancer. Think of every day and meal as an opportunity to make a healthy choice.

How do you recognize healthy eating patterns?

Tips for healthy eating

1. Base your meals on higher-fibre, starchy carbohydrates.

2. Eat lots of fruit and vegetables.

3. Eat more fish, including a portion of oily fish.

4. Cut down on saturated fat and sugar.

5. Eat less salt: no more than 6g a day for adults.

6. Get active and maintain a healthy weight.

7. Do not get thirsty.

8. Do not skip breakfast.

Diet patterns that can boost longevity and cut chronic disease

Physicians have long encouraged patients to eat more whole grains, fruits, vegetables, nuts, and legumes to improve their health and control their weight.

The foundation of the longevity diet

- A legume- and whole-grain-rich pescatarian or vegetarian diet

- 30% of calories come from vegetable fats such as nuts and olive oil.

- A low but sufficient protein diet until age 65, and then moderate protein intake

- Low-sugar and refined carbs

- No red or processed meat.

- Limited white meat.

Researchers analyzed hundreds of studies to identify a diet that optimizes human health and longevity.

They found that diets low in animal protein and high in complex carbohydrates that include periods of fasting are most beneficial for long-term health and life.

However, the researchers note that their findings simply provide a foundation for understanding and that, in practice, diets should be tailored to individual needs and circumstances.

However, what precisely makes up the optimal diet remains controversial. Growing evidence suggests optimal diets may depend on an interplay of health factors, including age, sex, and genetics.

The foundation of the longevity diet

For the study, the researchers analyzed hundreds of studies examining nutrition and delayed aging in short-lived species, nutrient response pathways, caloric restriction, fasting, and diets with various macronutrient and composition levels, such as the keto diet.

The studies analyzed nutrition and diet from multiple angles, from cellular and animal studies to clinical and epidemiological research investigating the lifestyles of centenarians.

In the end, the researchers found that the 'longevity diet includes:

- A legume and whole grain-rich pescatarian or vegetarian diet

- 30% of calories come from vegetable fats such as nuts and olive oil.

- A low but sufficient protein diet until age 65, and then moderate protein intake

- Low-sugar and refined carbs

- No red or processed meat

- Limited white meat

- 12 hours of eating and 12 hours of fasting per day

- Around three cycles of a five-day fasting-mimicking diet per year

Nutrition tips for better health and longevity

Following these nutrition tips will help a person make healthy food choices.

1. **Include protein with every meal.**

Including some protein with every meal can help balance blood sugar.

Higher-protein diets can be beneficial for type 2 diabetes.

Balancing blood sugar can support weight management and cardiovascular health.

2. Eat oily fish.

Omega-3 fatty acids in oily fish are essential for cell signaling, gene expression, and brain and eye development.

Omega-3 fatty acids can reduce the risk of cardiovascular disease.

The anti-inflammatory properties of omega-3 may effectively manage the early stages of degenerative diseases such as Alzheimer's disease and Parkinson's disease.

3. Eat whole grains.

Whole grains contain nutrients such as B vitamins, iron, and fiber. These nutrients are essential for body functions that include carrying oxygen in the blood, regulating the immune system, and balancing blood sugar.

4. Eat a rainbow.

The saying 'eat a rainbow' helps remind people to eat different colored fruits and vegetables.

Varying the color of plant foods means that someone gets a wide variety of antioxidants beneficial to health, for example, carotenoids and anthocyanins.

5. Eat your greens.

Dark green leafy vegetables are a great source of nutrition.

Leafy greens are rich in vitamins, minerals, and antioxidants.

The folate in leafy greens may help protect against cancer, while vitamin K helps prevent osteoporosis.

6. Include healthy fats.

People should limit their intake of saturated fats.

A person can replace these fats with unsaturated fats, which they can find in foods such as avocados, oily fish, and vegetable oils.

7. Use extra virgin olive oil.

As part of the Mediterranean diet, extra virgin olive oil has benefits for the heart, blood pressure, and weight.

A person can include extra virgin olive oil in their diet by adding it to salads or vegetables or cooking food at low temperatures.

8. Eat nuts

Eating one serving of nuts daily in place of red or processed meat, French fries, or dessert may benefit health and prevent long-term weight gain.

The AHA suggests that Brazil nuts, in particular, may help someone feel fuller and stabilize their blood sugar.

9. Get enough Fibre.

Fibre can help improve blood cholesterol levels and lower the risk of heart disease, obesity, and type 2 diabetes.

People can get enough fiber in their diet by eating whole grains, vegetables, beans, and pulses.

10. Increase plant foods.

Plant-based diets may help prevent overweight and obesity. Doctors associate obesity with many diseases.

According to some studies, including more plant foods in the diet could increase the risk of developing diseases such as diabetes and cardiovascular disease.

11. Try beans and pulses.

Beans and pulses are a good source of protein for people on a plant-based diet. However, those who eat meat can eat it on a few meat-free days a week.

Beans and pulses also contain beneficial fibre, vitamins, and minerals.

Pulses may help people feel fuller and lose Nutritional tips for what to drink

Drinking plenty of healthy fluids has numerous health benefits. Health experts recommend these tips:

12. Drink water

Drinking enough water every day is good for overall health and can help manage body weight. Drinking water can prevent dehydration. If someone does not like plain water, they can add some citrus slices and mint leaves to increase the appeal or drink herbal teas.

13. Enjoy coffee

A 2017 study suggests that moderate coffee consumption of 3–5 cups a day can reduce the risk of:

- type 2 diabetes

- Alzheimer's disease

- Parkinson's disease

- cardiovascular diseases

According to the same review, the recommended amount is reduced to 2 cups per day for pregnant and lactating people.

14. Drink herbal teas.

Catechins in green, black, and other herbal teas may have antimicrobial properties.

Herbal teas, such as mint, chamomile, and rooibos, are caffeine-free and help keep someone hydrated throughout the day.

Nutrition tips for foods and drinks to avoid

It is important to cut back on foods and drinks that may have harmful health consequences. For example, a person may want to:

15. Reduce sugar

Dietary sugar, dextrose, and high fructose corn syrup may increase the risk of cardiovascular disease and metabolic syndrome.

People should look out for hidden sugars in foods that manufacturers label as names ending in "-ose," for example, fructose, sucrose, and glucose.

Natural sugars, such as honey and maple syrup, could also contribute to weight gain if someone eats them too often.

16. Drink alcohol in moderation.

If someone consumes alcohol, it should be in moderation.

They advise up to one drink per day for females and up to two drinks per day for males.

Excessive drinking increases the risk of chronic diseases and violence and, over time, can impair short- and long-term cognitive function.

17. Avoid sugary drinks.

Frequently drinking sugary drinks with:

- weight gain and obesity
- type 2 diabetes
- heart disease
- kidney disease
- non-alcoholic liver disease
- tooth decay and cavities
- gout, a type of arthritis

People should limit their consumption of sugary drinks and, preferably, drink water instead.

18. Eat less red and processed meat.

U.S. adults eating more red and processed meat had higher mortality rates.

Participants who swapped meat for other protein sources, such as fish, nuts, and eggs, had a lower risk of death in the eight-year study period.

19. Avoid processed foods.

According to a review in Nutrients, eating ultra-processed foods can increase the risk of many diseases, including cancer, irritable bowel syndrome, and depression.

People should instead consume whole foods and avoid foods with long lists of processed ingredients.

Other good health habits

There are several steps a person can take to improve their health in addition to consuming healthy foods and drinks.

20. Support your microbiome.

A 2019 review in Nutrients a high-quality, balanced diet supports microbial diversity and can influence the risk of chronic diseases.

The authors indicate that including vegetables and fiber is beneficial to the microbiome. Conversely, eating too many refined carbohydrates and sugars is detrimental.

21. Consider a vitamin D supplement.

The recommended dietary allowance for vitamin D is 15 micrograms, or 600 international units per day, for adults.

Many people get some of their vitamin D from sunlight, while it is also in some foods.

People with darker skin, older adults, and those who get less exposure to sunlight—

such as during the winter or in less sunny climates—may need to take a vitamin D supplement.

22. be aware of portion sizes.

Being aware of portion sizes can help people manage their weight and diet.

People can adapt the guidelines to suit their cultural or personal preferences.

23. Use herbs and spices.

Using herbs and spices in cooking can liven up a meal and have additional health benefits.

The active compounds in ginger may help prevent oxidative stress and inflammation that occur as part of aging.

Curcumin in turmeric is anti-inflammatory and may have protective effects on health. Garlic has many benefits. Including anti-inflammatory, antimicrobial, and antioxidant properties.

23. Give your body a rest by fasting.

Intermittent fasting involves not eating either overnight or some days of the week. This may reduce energy intake and have health benefits. Intermittent fasting may improve blood pressure, cholesterol levels, and heart health.

24. Keep a food journal.

The American Society for Nutrition says that keeping a food journal can help people track calories, see how much they are eating, and recognize food habits.

Keeping a food journal could help someone who wants to maintain a moderate weight or eat a more healthy diet.

25. Wash fruits and vegetables.

Raw fruits and vegetables can contain harmful germs that could make someone sick. According to research, *Salmonella, E.*

coli, and *Listeria* cause a large percentage of U.S. foodborne illnesses.

Always wash fresh produce when eating it raw.

26. Do not microwave in plastic containers.

Microwaving food in plastic containers can release phthalates, which can disrupt hormones.

Experts recommend heating food in glass or ceramic containers that are microwave-safe.

27. Eat varied meals.

Many people eat the same meals regularly. Varying foods and trying different cuisines can help someone achieve their required nutrient intake.

This can be particularly helpful when trying to eat a broader range of vegetables or protein.

28. Eat mindfully

Mindful eating helps adults with obesity eat fewer sweets and manage their blood glucose.

Another study by Trusted Source suggests mindfulness can bring greater awareness to food triggers and habits in people with diabetes.

Simple Ways to Adopt a Healthy, Sustainable Eating Pattern

Changing your dietary habits can be hard, but with meal planning, lifestyle adjustments, and mindful eating practices, you can succeed. Consider consulting a nutritionist or doctor for the best approach.

In today's dynamic and fast-paced world, sticking to a healthy diet is sometimes easier said than done. Most of us know the feeling.

For starters, just sifting through the array of healthy diets to figure out which one is best for you can be a challenge.

But even after you've picked out a meal plan or eating pattern, maintaining that healthy diet day in and day out has its fair share of difficulties.

The good news is, no matter how tough it might feel some days, sticking to a healthy diet is possible, and it doesn't even mean that you have to give up your favorite foods.

There are tons of tips and tricks that make eating healthy easier, and most of them are simple and free.

Here are 11 of our favorite ways to stick to a healthy diet.

1. **Eat a diet rich in whole foods.**

There are many ways to follow a healthy diet, and no two nutritious diets look the same.

Still, most successful, long-term healthy diets have at least one thing in common: they're rich in whole foods.

Whole foods are those that have been minimally processed, such as:

- fruits

- vegetables

- legumes

- whole grains

- nuts and seeds

- eggs and dairy

- fresh animal proteins

Shakes, supplements, and fad diets might seem useful on the surface, but time and time again, whole-food diets have been linked to better health outcomes all around the world.

Whole foods are high in fibre, vitamins, minerals, and phytonutrients that support a healthy gut and reduce the risk of chronic diseases like obesity and diabetes.

On the contrary, ultra-processed foods like chips, candy, and sodas are more likely to promote inflammation and encourage chronic diseases.

2. Think twice before you crash a diet.

One of the most important questions to ask yourself when starting a healthy diet is, "Can I keep this up long-term?"

If the answer to that question is no, you could be embarking on a crash diet.

Crash diets usually rely on extreme calorie restriction to obtain fast weight loss results.

But here's the thing about crash diets—actually, the thing about diets in general, from keto to Atkins and everything in between—the results usually don't last in the long run. Over time, most people who diet regain the weight they've lost.

Interestingly, one diet that has held up to the test of time is the Mediterranean diet, and it's rich in whole foods.

Thus, when it comes to sticking with a healthy diet, try to resist the urge to focus too much on weight loss.

Oftentimes, the healthy habits you instill by eating a nutritious diet end up being more important in the long run than how much weight you've lost in a short period.

3. **Lean on professionals to get started.**

Simply put, adopting a healthy diet can be intimidating and challenging.

There are so many diets to choose from that you may feel like you don't even know where to start. It seems like everyone under the sun has an opinion on what you should and shouldn't eat.

The good news is that you aren't alone on this journey.

Many trained professionals can help you figure out the best path for you.

A registered dietitian can help you navigate meal plans, food groups, your daily nutrient needs, and safe diets for specific conditions and diseases.

A behavior change specialist, such as a psychologist, can help you break old habits and form new ones.

4. **Learn the right diet for you.**

It's not uncommon to hear about diets described as being the "best" or "healthiest."

Yet, no one diet works best for everyone.

We each live in a unique set of circumstances influenced by genetics, our health, work schedules, family, cultural traditions, and more.

No single diet can perfectly account for or accommodate so many individual factors.

In the end, the "best" healthy diet for you is the one that makes you feel your best and that you can stick with for the long haul.

5. **Surround yourself with healthy foods.**

In recent years, researchers have found that people around the world are eating more ultra-processed foods than ever before.

Ultra-processed foods are those that have been made by industrial processing. They tend to contain additives like sweeteners, thickeners, stabilizers, and other ingredients that make the foods last longer and taste better.

Some examples of ultra-processed foods include fast food, frozen dinners, and sugar-sweetened juices and sodas.

Not only are ultra-processed foods tempting due to their flavors, but even being in the presence of these types of foods can affect brain chemistry and behavior.

You can help avoid the temptation to eat these foods by keeping them out of your house and limiting your access to them at home.

On the other hand, keeping your fridge and pantry stocked with nutrient-dense, whole foods is a great way to keep your healthy diet in mind and encourage yourself to have those nutritious foods more often.

6. **Keep filling snacks on hand.**

Often, it's the moments when we find ourselves feeling extra hungry and tempted by a tasty treat that we forget about the healthy eating plans we had in mind for the day.

Though craving foods from time to time is completely normal, researchers have found that in moments of extreme hunger, our cravings tend to get even stronger.

Keeping nutritious and <u>filling snacks</u> on hand is a great way to keep cravings at bay until your next full meal.

Snacks that are high in protein and fibre can help keep you feeling full.

Some examples are:

- fresh fruits and veggies

- yoghurt

- popcorn

- hard-boiled eggs

- mixed nuts and nut butter

- Hummus or roasted chickpeas

- whole-grain crackers

7. Save your favorite foods.

- Have you ever felt like there's one food you just can't live without? Fortunately, you don't have to!

- Depriving yourself of the foods you love and crave can end up backfiring.

- In the short term, it tends to make your cravings for those foods even stronger, especially for people who are more susceptible to food cravings in general.

- Some research has even found that feeling satisfied rather than deprived while dieting is linked to a higher rate of weight loss.

- Rather than completely giving up the less nutritious foods that you love, try having them only occasionally while practicing portion control.

8. Avoid an all-or-nothing approach.

- A common barrier people encounter while working towards improving their diets is falling into an all-or-nothing mindset.

- An all-or-nothing thought might sound something like this: "Well, I've already ruined my diet for the day by having that piece of cake at the office party earlier, so I might as well forget my plans to cook at home tonight and grab takeout instead."

- These types of thoughts usually look at situations in black and white, or as "good" and "bad."

- Instead, try to look at each food choice you make during the day as its own. One less-than-ideal choice doesn't have to snowball into a full day's worth of similar choices.

- In fact, having high self-esteem and confidence in your ability to make healthy choices tends to be associated with better health outcomes, so don't let one small stumble bring you down.

9. Plan for eating out.

For many people, potlucks, happy hours, and dining out is something to look forward to. But for someone struggling to stick to a new or healthy diet, it can feel like another hurdle to overcome.

Restaurant meals tend to be higher in calories, sodium, sugar, fat, and ultra-processed foods than meals cooked at home, and they often come in large serving sizes.

Plus, in social settings, our own food choices are heavily influenced by the choices of the people around us.

Simply put, it's easy to overdo it when eating out, and maintaining a healthy diet while eating out can be very challenging.

Still, there are ways to make it easier. Having a strategy in mind before you get to a restaurant or gathering can go a long way toward easing your mind and helping you feel prepared to navigate eating out.

Here are a few of our favorite tips for eating out:

- Research the menu before you go.
- Eat a piece of fruit ahead of time.
- Stay hydrated during the meal.
- Order your meal first.
- Take your time and eat your meal.

10. Monitor your progress.

Self-monitoring is an easy and effective way to keep track of your progress on your own.

It can be as simple as keeping a journal of the foods you eat each day or as detailed as using a smartphone or web-based app that tracks the details of your daily calorie intake, weight, activity levels, and more.

When self-monitoring your progress, remember that weight loss and gain are not the only ways to measure how far you've come. In some cases, they might not be the best way to measure progress either.

People choose to follow healthy diets for all types of different reasons. For example, you might choose to focus on how your dietary changes have affected your physical or mental health rather than how much weight you've lost.

Some other questions to ask yourself to help measure whether your healthier diet is working are:

- Am I full and satisfied?

- Do I enjoy what I eat?

- Could I keep eating this way forever?

- How many healthy choices did I make today?

- How confident do I feel about my diet?

- Have I noticed any changes to my physical health?

- Have I noticed any changes to my mental health?

11. Be patient with yourself.

- Sticking to a healthier diet is a marathon, not a sprint.

- Learning the best diet for yourself takes trial and error, and some days will be easier than others, so try not to feel discouraged if it takes longer than you'd like for your new habits to set in.

- As long as you set realistic expectations for yourself, remain committed, and continue to reevaluate your progress, your diet is likely to keep moving in a positive direction.

Chapter 4

The science of hunger and health

When do we feel hungry?

What is hunger?

Hunger is an uncomfortable or painful physical sensation caused by insufficient consumption of dietary energy. It becomes chronic when the person does not consume a sufficient amount of calories (dietary energy) regularly to lead a normal, active, and healthy life. For decades, FAO has used the prevalence of undernourishment indicator to estimate the extent of hunger in the world; thus, "hunger" may also be referred to as undernourishment.

 Hunger is a physical sensation experienced only when the body needs food. It may cause you to feel empty, or your stomach may rumble. "We typically throw this term around loosely when we want something to eat, not when we need something."

When your stomach is empty, it contracts or collapses, causing hunger pangs. Your blood sugar levels dip and your stomach produces a hormone called ghrelin, prompting you to eat. Psychological hunger: Psychological or emotional hunger is not caused by true physiological hunger or the need for nutrition.

It also affects muscle and organ function. People who are malnourished or go without food will feel overall weaker and more fatigued and experience sensations like lightheadedness and dizziness. Hunger also affects adult immune systems, making people more susceptible to disease.

What is food insecurity?

A person is food insecure when they lack regular access to enough safe and nutritious food for normal growth and development and an active and healthy life. This may be due to the unavailability of food and/or a lack of resources to obtain food. Food insecurity can be experienced at different levels of severity.

Why do we get hungry?

Hunger serves an obvious purpose: it tells us that we need to eat to keep our bodies fueled. Yet most of us live in a world where food is ever-present and meals are scheduled around social conventions. Do we need a reminder to eat breakfast, lunch, and dinner?

So. While our society may have evolved to provide us with endless opportunities to eat, our bodies are primarily concerned with keeping the well-oiled machine going.

This means that we start to feel hungry once our stomach is empty. However, the sighting of a tasty Halloween treat being shared in the office may tempt us, even though we're not technically hungry.

That's because our brains are on the lookout for energy-rich foods, just in case we need to go without them later on.

And the key word in this sentence is "brain," because our grey matter is in charge of hunger.

Hunger and an empty stomach

After a meal, our gastrointestinal tracts slowly empty by pushing food through the stomach and the small and large intestines.

Specialized contractions called the migrating motor complex (MMC) sweep up undigested food, which is a process that takes around 130 minutes. The final phase of the MMC is regulated by a hormone called motilin. Motilin-controlled contractions cause the rumbling in our stomachs and coincide with those in humans.

Another hormone implicated in hunger control is ghrelin. In mice, ghrelin neurons called agouti-related peptide (AgRP) expression neurons in the hypothalamus region of the brain tell us that we are hungry.

These neurons are the control center for hunger. When AgRP neurons are artificially switched on in mice, they gorge themselves on food.

So, our brains pick up messages from our stomachs and tell us that it's time for our next meal, around 2 hours after we've eaten. But that doesn't explain the irresistible draw of a delicious snack between meals.

Appealing snacks and the brain

Here, we need to differentiate between homeostatic hunger, which is related purely to balancing our short-term energy reserves, and hedonic hunger, which makes use of opportunities to gather extra energy. Hedonic hunger is less well understood than homeostatic hunger.

When our eyes detect something that we have previously enjoyed eating, our brain is notified.

If we are full, we might take a rain check. However, our brains are hardwired to avoid running out of energy. The offer of extra food can therefore override our feeling of fullness and lead us to grab that tasty snack after all.

How we feel about our previous meal may also have something to do with it.

Medical News Today recently reported on a study that showed that participants who were under the impression that they had eaten a smaller breakfast ate a larger lunch and had more daily calories than those who thought that they had eaten a bigger breakfast.

Hunger and overeating

So, our brains control our hunger based on what we eat, whether or not we feel that what we've eaten is enough to make us full, and the availability of extra calories.

This system may have worked while humans were hunter-gatherers, but these days, it contributes to overeating and the steady rise of obesity.

Maintaining a healthy diet and weight may therefore be a battle between what we tell our brains and what our brains tell us. In that spirit, I've decided to opt for the more healthful Halloween treats.

Hunger 'seems to override' satiety.

All of the participants were given blood samples and completed questionnaires about their feelings of hunger and fullness 4 weeks, 1 year, and 2 years after the start of the program. From the blood samples, the team was able to assess levels of hormones that control hunger and fullness, or satiety.

The participants did not report a change in their feelings of fullness at the 4-week assessment but did report a reduction after 1 and 2 years of sustained weight loss. In contrast, they reported a significant increase in hunger at the 1- and 2-year assessments.

The blood tests showed higher levels of both satiety and hunger hormones after 1 and 2 years of sustained weight loss.

How a protein helps with weight loss

The food you eat provides you with energy in the form of calories.

There are three basic forms that these calories can take: carbohydrates, fats, and protein.

The protein leverage hypothesis essentially proposes that when you don't consume enough protein, you'll feel hungry, even if you're getting calories from other sources.

"Basically, when you don't eat enough calories from protein in comparison to calories from carbs and fat, you end up eating more calories in an attempt to meet those minimum protein requirements and can often end up overeating in general," she explained.

The relevance of protein leverage tends to be increased in highly industrialized areas of the world, including the United States, where processed foods high in sugar (a carbohydrate) and fat are often more affordable and readily available than fresh foods.

How to increase protein in your diet

In theory, protein leverage could be a useful concept both as a tool and as a potentially avoidable obstacle to managing weight loss and maintaining a healthy weight.

For example, by intentionally consuming protein, you might be able to avoid feelings of hunger that could otherwise lead to overeating.

"One could prevent [protein leverage] from contributing to obesity by prioritizing protein-rich foods at meal and snack times, aiming for balanced meals, staying hydrated, and managing portion sizes," she explained.

In addition to those strategies, when eating grains, choosing ones that are whole grains will increase the protein and fibre content. This advice might help you maintain a healthy weight or avoid weight gain again, but how might protein leverage be a factor if you're trying to lose weight?

Losing weight means cutting calories, and if those calories come from protein, then that person may very well end up eating more and therefore curbing their weight loss.

However, this doesn't mean that protein should be your exclusive source of caloric intake, as this could lead to other negative health consequences.

How can protein impact obesity?

The review paper notes that there is no single cause of obesity.

The authors say that the protein leverage hypothesis is only one potential factor among others that range from the genetic to the behavioral, cultural, and even geopolitical.

There is never one answer to eating concerns, but protein is a critical nutrient and very directly related to satiety, strength, immune health, and healthy weight, so prioritizing protein at meals and snacks is a good idea for many reasons.

But protein leverage itself can be complex, as protein requirements can be different from person to person and even vary over your life.

Weight loss is not working.

You may find that after your initial weight loss, your progress will slow down and eventually stop. Some common reasons for plateaus include: doing the same workouts over and over. Your body needs to be challenged to progress, so make sure you're changing some part of your program every four to six weeks.

When a person wants to lose weight, trying inappropriate diet and exercise routines is a common mistake.

Calories are a unit of measure that shows the amount of energy in foods and drinks. The body requires a certain number of calories to function.

It will convert any excess calories into fat, increasing overall weight. The body can only lose weight when it burns more calories than it takes in.

A person can lose weight through a calorie-restricted diet and regular physical activity. However, many factors can prevent weight loss.

Learn How Hunger Works to Avoid Getting Hangry

You walk into a restaurant. You're famished. It's in your eyes and growling loudly from your stomach. Once hunger hits, it can't be reversed until you eat. The beast must be satisfied. And the server knows it from how quickly your eyes devour the menu and lock in on an order.

It's easy for objectivity, rationality, and patience to go out the window as your body takes over. Your stomach—and brain, for that matter—kick start several processes that motivate you to fill your face with food as quickly as possible.

You know what's to blame for the hunger. But what else is going on behind the scenes, deep within your body's appetite control center? It's time to find out.

Blame your hunger hormones.

Hunger can seem to strike out of nowhere. But it starts with the flip of a switch that fires up the neuronal network in your brain— mainly within the hypothalamus. These nerve cells within the hypothalamus are gatekeepers for your brain. They're the key to allowing the body to communicate and interpret hunger cues.

Depending on whether you're hungry or full, these nerve cells either receive or block signals from various hormones. The two main hunger hormones are ghrelin and leptin, and insulin plays a role a little later on in the process.

When your stomach is empty, it sends ghrelin onto a pathway from the gut to the brain. Ghrelin is the message handed from your gut to your brain, saying, "It's time to eat." So, allowing signals from ghrelin released from the stomach to communicate with the hypothalamus increases appetite. Once you start to eat, ghrelin production begins to back off.

Leptin is ghrelin's opposing force—hunger's off switch. This hormone, which originates in fat cells, decreases hunger when it's allowed to talk to the brain. It's the signal your fat cells send when they have enough energy from a meal. And it tells your brain it's time to stop shoveling food into your mouth.

The decision to block or allow entry happens at the opening of the blood-brain barrier of the hypothalamus. This area is an entry point where hormones released by the gut, pancreas, and fat cells (also called adipose tissue) can pass through to communicate with the brain.

It's not a one-way street, though. Hormones secreted from the hypothalamus use this portal as an exit, traveling in the opposite direction out into the body. This dance between hunger hormones—and those signals originating in your brain—is what balances your hunger and impacts your body's energy reserves, weight, and body composition.

As you digest, your hunger steadily decreases. That's because leptin—and its appetite-diminishing effects—gain prominence. Insulin (another important hormone that helps carry energy to cells) decreases rapidly. This also helps suppress appetite. So after you eat, insulin and leptin team up to inhibit hunger and help bring about a feeling of satiety.

Save the Day, Keep Hanger at Bay

A busy day, congested traffic, and an overflowing email inbox there are so many reasons you find yourself at the intersection of Hungry and Angry—better known as Hangry.

It's not a place you choose to visit. And as soon as you arrive at Hangry, you're desperate to leave. That's because hunger and the accompanying irritability are intensely unpleasant, uncomfortable, and unwelcome for you and anyone in your immediate vicinity.

While "hangry" is a newer word, coined to lend humor to an otherwise annoying situation, the hanger can be very real. Scientists agree there is biological and psychological validity to the state of hunger. One nutritionist, Sophie Medlin, even claims it is a bona fide emotion.

But what's going on? Hunger isn't always accompanied by an emotional meltdown, so what brings about this extra reaction? Researchers at the University of North Carolina at Chapel Hill found two factors determine hangers: context and self-awareness. The researchers conducted two studies to demonstrate this.

In the first experiment, participants were primed for a specific mood by viewing curated images associated with positive, neutral, or negative emotions. The images were shown to induce the corresponding mood. Immediately after priming, the participants were shown an ambiguous image and asked to rate it. The participants were also asked to evaluate how hungry they felt.

Results showed that after viewing negative images, hungrier participants were more likely to rate the ambiguous image as negative. The participants projected their negative feelings of hunger onto their subjective assessment of the image. Having a somewhat negative experience while hungry can skew your perceptions, making you report the image as more intensely negative. So, context matters.

The second experiment explored the other influential factor of hangers: self-awareness. Researchers required half of the participants to fast beforehand. The other half could eat as they normally would. Some participants were then asked to complete an assignment in which they reflected on and wrote about their emotions.

Then all participants were given a tiresome computer task. During the activity, the program underwent a planned crash to evoke frustration. Study coordinators blamed the crash on the participants to further rile them up. Lastly, all participants were asked to fill out a survey to evaluate their experience and identify their emotions.

Researchers found that fast participants who did not reflect on and write about their emotions before the computer task reported more negative feelings. They even reported feeling hateful towards the coordinators, who blamed them for the computer crash. The results demonstrated that emotional self-awareness plays a part in being hungry.

So, if you're aware of your intense hunger as it builds, you're less likely to view it as a negative emotional experience. Alternatively, if you neglect to check in with your emotions and you become hungry, you're more likely to lash out in frustration at a frustrating situation.

Get Ahead of Hunger, Ride out Satiety

Just because being hungry is a real possibility doesn't mean you need to experience it. Arm yourself with tools and plan to avoid excessive hunger—and potential hunger—

altogether. There are three important steps you can take today.

1. Understand the Glycemic Index

A glycemic index is a value assigned to a food based on how quickly your body can convert the food into usable energy, or glucose. Simple carbohydrates (think refined sugar or white bread) will fall on the high end of the glycemic index. That's because the energy within them is readily available for use by the body. More complex carbohydrates, like whole grains and vegetables, release glucose slowly and steadily, so they fall on the low end of the index. It's because they have more fibre to slow down the digestion process.

Those are the basics. You can dive deeper if you want, but you should be familiar enough with this concept to use it to your advantage! Here are some ideas.

- Reach for foods on the low end of the glycemic index. These foods take longer to break down, meaning you avoid a quick spike of energy followed by a crash. That's because low-glycemic foods provide you with more sustained energy over time.

- Pair high-glycemic foods with something on the lower end. For example, if you're having a carb-heavy meal, add a colorful side salad. Skip the hearts of romaine and go for deeper greens. Spruce up the salad with other colorful veggies like bell peppers, carrots, or beets. The veggie boost will provide a healthy dose of fibre to help slow down the digestion of the simpler carbs. Or add some healthy fats or protein to further delay carb digestion.

2. **Start your day right.**

As you've probably heard, breakfast is very important. When you skip breakfast, you're almost asking for a one-way ticket to Hangry Town. Keep your belly full and your mind sharp by having a balanced meal to start the day. If your mornings are busy, consider packing a healthy snack the night before. Then, if hunger creeps up before lunchtime, you have a go-to hanger stopper within reach.

3. **Protein is anti-hangry.**

Protein helps keep you feeling fuller for longer. So, it's a great idea to examine what kinds of meals and snacks you normally eat. If you find your meals short on, or completely devoid of, protein, get creative.

- Don't assume that protein means meat. There are many meat alternatives on the market. Whether it's tofu, seitan, tempeh, or a mix of veggie proteins, the options are plentiful. If these alternative proteins are new to you, read up and consider adding one or two to your diet for some variety.

- If you are a meat eater, vary your sources. Consider a new type of meat or fish. If you already eat a variety, switch up how it's prepared. For example, if you enjoy turkey, ask your butcher to grind it and make your burger patties. Your market should be staffed by butchers well-versed in different cuts, preparation styles, and even recipe ideas. If not, there are ways to accomplish these tasks at home.

- Pair a healthy midday snack, like carrots, apples, or celery, with nut butter. It can give you the perfect mix of savory and sweet while also providing you with a serving of protein.

If these tips are new to you, start slow. If you're overzealous, you may find that the new habits are harder to adopt. Instead, pick out one that feels doable and start there. Once you've incorporated a new habit successfully, try adding another to the mix.

How do our bodies control appetite?

Appetite regulation is the system that governs appetite, which means the processes taking place in our body that result in us feeling hungry or full. This is an extremely complicated and integrated system that regulates around 1 million calories our bodies consume throughout the year. Even when a little weight is gained throughout this period, it takes an incredibly efficient system to perform such a balancing act of calories in and calories out.

How does our appetite regulation system work?

The role of our brain

The brain is important in this appetite regulation system, especially a section that's so deeply ingrained called the hypothalamus. The hypothalamus is the feeding center and is responsible for numerous different homeostatic processes; one such process is keeping our body in a balanced state, like feeding and fasting, for example. The hypothalamus releases different hormones to make us feel full or hungry. These signals depend entirely on what's happening lower down in the body—our gut!

The role of our gut

Throughout the gut are cells called enter endocrine cells, which sense the environment and then send a message to the brain to release an appetite-stimulating hormone or an appetite-suppressing hormone after indulging in a breakfast buffet, for example, these cells will sense the large volume of food consumed and signal to the brain to suppress appetite. Or, after a day without eating, these same cells will release a hunger hormone to signal the brain to feel hungry and consume food.

When losing weight or simply trying to take our minds off food, staying full and satisfied is essential. Let's take a quick look at some of the tricks we can do to feel fuller throughout the day.

Food choices that help us stay fuller for longer

Fibre: is the structure of plant-based foods and is indigestible, which means we can't digest fibre and use it for energy; it contains no calories. It is found in numerous plant-based food groups, and you'll find the highest quantities of fiber in:

Non-starchy vegetables: spinach, kale, broccoli, asparagus

Seeds and nuts: flaxseeds, chia seeds, almonds, and cashews

Beans and pulses: lentils, black beans, chickpeas

Research has shown these enter endocrine cells receive signals from fiber to release hormones that signal to the brain to make us feel fuller. Although the exact quantity of fiber needed to produce these effects isn't yet known, there does seem to be more and more evidence highlighting its appetite-suppressing qualities.

Protein is an essential part of a healthy, balanced diet, and you may be aware of its role in muscle recovery, but it's also quite a potent appetite suppressor! Protein is digested more slowly compared to carbohydrates, a process termed 'delayed gastric emptying'. It has been shown to elevate hormones that suppress our appetite, leading to increased feelings of fullness (5). High-quality protein sources include:

- Meat and poultry

- Fish

- Dairy

- Tofu

- Legumes

Chapter 5

How to learn to love sleep

How Do You Get Enough Sleep? Here's How Many Hours You Need

How important is sleep, why should you care, and how will improper sleep hygiene mess with your health and wellness?

Want to know how to sleep better? You're not alone.

We're not sleeping enough, and it's killing us.

As a nation, we're the most exhausted, overworked, and under-rested bunch in history. It's bad for our health, for our looks, and for our work performance.

70 million US adults suffer from sleep loss every day. We spend over $66 billion on sleep medication, devices, and clinical visits, and fractured sleep time costs over $411 billion every year.

Worse, cheating on sleep will not give you a long and healthy life. The overwhelming body of scientific sleep research shows sleep loss promotes cardiovascular disease, dementia, and death.

But we can't just work less, "have less stress," and meditate two hours a day. That would be wonderful and practical if we were rich like Gwyneth Paltrow.

The good news? We can take steps to fix sleep problems, but there's no one-size-fits-all solution. The real cure for all those 3 a.m. angst sessions is pinpointing the exact cause of your sleeplessness and then taking a targeted approach.

In this article, we'll look at the many causes of sleep loss that torpedo work performance, health, and productivity. We'll see fixes from apps to medications to sleep tips used by Navy SEALs to fall asleep in seconds. In the process, we'll hear from bona fide sleep experts who've helped millions get the deep, restful sleep patterns we crave and need.

Why do we need to switch our brains off for 8 hours every night? Sleep time lets us rest, restore, and repair, and it may even keep our brains young and "plastic." Understanding the importance of sleep is a key step in knowing how to sleep better.

Brain plasticity; a brain can get "stiff" like an unused muscle. Harvard Medical School research shows knowing how to sleep better can improve focus, learning, mood, and decision-making ability.

Restoration. Human and animal studies show sleep restores, rejuvenates, and repairs our minds and bodies. Animals deprived of sleep entirely die in a matter of weeks when their immune systems collapse. Sleep aids in tissue repair and muscle growth. It also clears the brain of amyloid plaques found in Alzheimer's patients.

Energy conservation. During sleep time, our metabolisms drop. In the modern world, plentiful food supplies make that less of a survival matter and more of a carbon footprint issue. In short, 8 billion people who never slept would consume the planet's resources at a faster rate.

Safety. Researchers once thought of sleep as a safety issue. Sleeping in the dark may have kept us safe from nighttime predators like tigers. This theory has been discredited because it would be safer to stay still *and* conscious than to fall asleep.

The Dangers of Losing Sleep

Why is sleep important? When you don't sleep, the world becomes a living nightmare. Things that seem petty in daylight turn monstrous. Worse, you know that without sleep, you'll be less well-equipped to solve those problems when the sun comes up.

But you're not alone. 70 million Americans suffer from sleeplessness every night. The costs of poor sleep patterns hit us at work, in our wallets, in our private lives, and in our health. Here are six big reasons to focus on how to sleep better.

1. $411billionninlfinancial Costs

How important is sleep to the economy? Accordingly, we lose 2–3% of global GDP to sleeplessness. That's $411 billion in lost productivity in the US alone. But even small changes to our sleep habits could have a massive impact. If everyone slept at least six hours a night, we'd add an estimated $226.4 billion to the US economy.

2. Lost Productivity: Why is sleep important? People in the US lose 1.2 million work days per year from a lack of sleep time.

3. Sleep loss risks in careers

How important is sleep to your career? Regularly missing sleep slashes concentration, reaction time, memory, and decision-making power. It crushes your interpersonal skills, one of the biggest determinants of career success.

Lack of sleep also causes accidents. Sleep loss was a contributing factor in disasters.

Like the Three Mile Island nuclear meltdown, the Exxon Valdez oil spill, and the Challenger Space Shuttle explosion. Tired workers are similar to drunk employees in terms of motor function, speech, memory, decision-making, and problem-solving.

Fatigue causes an estimated 100,000 car crashes per year.

Plus, as we move up the company ladder, we get both more responsibility and less sleep. The average senior manager and CEO get 25% less sleep time than the populace at large.

4. It wrecks your health

Want to live a long and healthy life? Learn how to sleep better. People who sleep less than six hours a night have a 13% higher chance of dying. What should keep you up at night, though (pun intended), is the variety of *ways* sleep loss wrecks your health. Here's a rundown:

- **Heart disease.** How important is sleep to your heart? Short-sleepers put themselves at a higher risk of dying from cardiovascular disease. Poor sleep patterns could be as dangerous to your heart as smoking.

- **Diabetes.** Obesity and type 2 diabetes are linked to short sleep durations. Possibly because short-sleepers eat more high-carb foods.

- **Alzheimer's disease and dementia** Cheat sleep, and your brain may suffer. "The brain needs deep REM sleep to prevent Alzheimer's disease," says sleep expert Walter Gaman, MD, of Executive Medicine of Texas. Alzheimer's disease is linked to the buildup of amyloid protein in the brain. Shockingly, even one night of missed sleep causes a 5% jump in brain amyloid.

- **Sex drive.** Need another reason to learn how to sleep better? Sleep deprivation causes sexual dysfunction as the brain suppresses sex hormones. That's worse for women than for men.

- **Depression.** Studies show over two-thirds of depression patients suffer from a sleep disorder. Insomniacs are four times more likely to develop depression if their sleep problems aren't addressed. Poor sleep is also linked to bipolar disorder, anxiety, and ADHD.

- **Unhealthy skin.** Beauty sleep—it's real! Lack of sleep time can lead to skin malnourishment, breakouts, dark circles, and eye bags. Want to look older fast? Just stop getting at least 7 hours of sleep a night.

- **Inflammation.** The new watchword for all our health woes is "inflammation." It's the trigger for just about every health baddie in our lives—from heart disease to dementia to cancer and rheumatoid arthritis. Sleep loss creates inflammatory cytokines that throw our bodies out of whack.

Poor immune system. Sleep boosts your immune system. How? When we don't sleep enough, we're more likely to get sick. Also, if you're sick, a good night's rest will help you beat it faster.

The grain of salt the "good" news? Sleeping *too long* has also been associated with nearly every health risk on this list. In short, there's a sweet spot—your sleep schedule should be 7–9 hours every day.

5. Sleep loss wrecks relationships

How important is sleep to your love life? Not getting enough sleep wrecks marriages and friendships. According to neurologist Chris Winter, author of The Sleep Solution, sleepless people talk to their partners less and help out less with household chores.

Why is sleep important to relationships? Poor sleepers feel sadder and angrier—not conducive to romance. Fractured sleep patterns can even contribute to divorce. The upside? Married people know how to sleep better. That gives them a leg up on their single peers.

6. Sleep sharpens your mind and heart.

 When you hear about people waking up from sleep with an answer to an unsolved problem or an idea for a new invention, you can thank REM sleep time. During REM, the brain consolidates memories. That means it converts new experiences into long-term memories.

Sleep also smooths out our emotions. "REM sleep allows your amygdala to process negative emotions, in particular fear and stress," says Nichols. Less REM sleep can cause negative memories to pile up, which can spark depression.

There are over 70 different sleep disorders that may be stealing your beauty sleep. But you can't know how to sleep better until you know the cause. So, here are the top sleep disorders.

Insomnia is sleeplessness caused by stress, disease, anxiety, depression, drug or alcohol abuse, and certain medications.

- **Fragmented sleep** patterns happen when someone wakes up frequently at night. It can ramp up levels of cortisol, the stress and inflammation hormone.

- **Trouble falling asleep.** Some people have a hard time nodding off each night.

- **Restless leg syndrome** is an irresistible urge to move your arms and legs at night. It affects 10% of the population. To fight it, cut caffeine and alcohol and get more exercise.

- **Sleep apnea** is a throat blockage that causes snoring and stops breathing. It can lead to sleepiness and death. The most common treatment is a CPAP machine.

- **Sleepwalking** stops us physically from resting. Want to know how to sleep better with a sleepwalking problem? Cut down on liquids before bedtime.

- **Night terrors.** Some illnesses and medications can cause nighttime screaming and violent movements. Doctors treat night terrors with medication.

- **REM sleep behavior disorder** happens when people thrash around during REM sleep time. Medication is the common fix.

- **Teeth grinding.** Excessive anxiety and stress can cause nighttime teeth grinding. To fix it, don't chew gum or other non-food items during the day.

- **Narcolepsy.** Some people have a blurred line between sleep and wakefulness. They may fall asleep during high-stress situations. It's treated with medication.

- **Circadian rhythm problems** Daily biological rhythms synchronize our sleep schedule to hours of darkness. When those rhythms get unbalanced, you lose sleep. The treatment is more natural light, especially in the morning.

- **Nighttime muscle cramps.** Some sleepers wake frequently from leg cramps. The solution? Exercise, stretching, and B12, but see a doctor to rule out underlying conditions.

Even when we want to know how to sleep better, we often can't. Below are the top reasons for short sleep times and sleep deprivation.

Choice. We're not asking, Why is sleep important? "Our culture today equates sleep with weakness, not the biological necessity it is," says Terry Cralle. "We think if we're high achievers, we have to learn to power through with less sleep." However research shows that with good sleep patterns, we get more done in less time than when we cheat on sleep.

Daytime caffeine zaps your sleep at night, making you more tired the next day without it. "Everyone's a little different in their tolerance, but I see too many people in Starbucks late in the day," says Cralle.

Shift work can crush our sleep patterns by disrupting our circadian rhythms and depriving us of natural daylight.

Being a parent with a young child can disrupt your sleep for up to 6 years after the child is born.

Certain diseases, like Lyme disease, can rob you of your sleep and leave you groggy during waking hours.

Not enough daylight. If you spend most of your day inside, you won't feel sleepy at night, and you'll be groggy during the day.

Diet. Eating well isn't just good for your health. It also helps you sleep.

Tips for better sleep

Can't figure out how to sleep better? Below are the best techniques for getting better sleep, according to sleep experts and neurologists.

1. Keep the clocks out of your bedroom

What's the biggest change you can make to get more sleep? Don't look at the clock during sleeping hours, says sleep expert Terry Cralle. Without a clock, the "chore" of falling asleep goes away. You won't start doing math in your head and worrying about how little sleep you're getting. If your room is dark and cool and you're "in the dark" about how much sleep you've missed, you'll most often fall back to sleep soon.

2. Follow a sleep schedule.

One of the biggest reasons we don't sleep is that we don't *respect* it. "People say they only have time for 4-5 hours a night," says Cralle. "But that can be dangerous, with studies showing metabolic changes after just a few nights of short sleep."

I wondered, "When should I wake up?" Or, "What time should I go to bed?" Try to go to bed as close to the first full darkness as you can, and rise with the sun. Going to sleep at 9 p.m., 10 p.m., or 11 p.m. matters less than keeping the same sleep schedule every night.

Is 6 hours of sleep enough?

Getting 6 hours of sleep a night will sap your focus, moods, health, and well-being. Always get 7–9 hours of in-the-bed sleep time, even if you're awake for some of it. Even if you feel fine after six hours of sleep, your effectiveness suffers.

3. Get more daylight.

Numerous studies show getting more natural light is one of the top techniques for sleeping better. Yet we've got ever-brighter screens on laptops and phones. Those screens—and our brightly lit homes—are sending silent messages to our brains that say, "It's morning! Go to sleep 12 hours from now." Trying to override those messages can be like eating a 32-ounce porterhouse steak right after Thanksgiving dinner. Your body will say, "Nope."

The upside? One-third of US employees work from home at least sometime during the week. That gives us a tremendous opportunity to work on a porch, park bench, or in an outdoor cafe. In winter, sit near a window for a few hours in the morning.

4. Have coffee cut-off times

Tired of being tired? Try switching to decaf after 2 p.m. Even drinking coffee six hours before bedtime can rob you of sleep time.

5. Try Audiobooks

Listening to an audiobook can help you sleep. Turn the volume down and set the playback to its slowest speed. Then set a timer so it shuts off in an hour. Most phones can set a "stop playback" alarm.

6. Distraction Techniques

When your mind has a tricky "job to do," it stays alert. "Some people fall asleep better with a distraction," says Cralle. So, here are a few tips for how to sleep better with distractions:

The Navy SEAL Technique

Why is sleep important for Navy SEALs? Imagine trying to sleep in the rain, in the cold, or in a fire zone when your life depends on being rested. Thankfully, these hardened warriors have a trick that helps them drift off in two minutes.

How to fall asleep:

1. Sit on the edge of your bed.

2. Relax the muscles of your face, jaw, tongue, and eyes.

3. Let your shoulders and arm muscles go slack.

4. Breathe out. Relax your chest, then your thighs, calves, feet, and toes.

5. Clear your mind for 10 seconds.

6. Picture one of these three images:

.You're lying in a pit room in a black velvet hammock.

.You're in a canoe on a calm lake with a blue sky above.

.You repeat the words "don't think" for 10 seconds.

The 2-minute Navy SEAL sleep technique works for 96% of sleepers. The downside? It can take six weeks of practice.

7. Meditation and meditation naps

Meditation can teach you how to sleep better by reducing stress. Here are a few meditation apps that can help you get your 40 winks:

Insight Timer is the #1 free meditation app for Android. 4.8 stars for 43K ratings.

Simple Habit Daily Meditation is a free meditation app for busy people.

"I like meditation," says neurologist Chris Winter. "When you start getting good at it and settling your mind, it becomes easier to fall asleep." And even if you don't learn how to sleep better, you still get good-quality mental rest.

8. Mantras, Prayers, Breathing, and Mandalas

Here are a few more relaxation and distraction techniques that can take your mind off: "I can't get to sleep!"

Mantras. A mantra may sound like money, but it's just a word or phrase you think repeatedly. How does it help you sleep? By filling your mind with something other than your worries,

Prayers. Same as mantras. Bonus: They get you in touch with your spiritual side.

Breathing techniques. When you focus on your breathing, you're distracted from the "chore" of trying to sleep. A great "how to sleep better" technique

Mandalas. A mandala is an image you imagine. It distracts you and helps you meditate or fall asleep. It can be a flower, a drawing, or even a stop sign.

9. Eat Well

Eating a healthy, balanced diet can improve your sleep time. Foods that impact tryptophan, serotonin, and melatonin, like eggs, cheese, and salmon, can help your sleep quality and duration.

Plus, take a magnesium supplement." Magnesium facilitates sleep-regulating melatonin production. Magnesium helps your sleep patterns and enhances memory.

10. Exercise

Daily exercise will help you fall asleep faster and stay asleep longer. But shouldn't you limit exercise before bed? New studies say exercising at any time of day will help you sleep. "I'd rather see people get some exercise than none because exercise begets quality sleep."

Stags of sleep; is sleep important?

The sleep cycle is the pattern of sleep stages from NREM (non-REM) to REM sleep (rapid eye movement). Each sleep cycle lasts 90 to 120 minutes and includes about 15 minutes of the four stages of sleep, including stages 1, 2, 3, and REM sleep.

- **Stage 1:** Light sleep; easy to wake. 5–10 min.

- **Stage 2:** Light sleep, preparing for deep sleep 10–15 min.

- **Stage 3:** Deep sleep It was hard to wake up. The body repairs itself and boosts the immune system.

- **REM sleep.** Rapid eye movements. Your brain clears plaques at this stage. 10 minutes to 1 hour. REM cycles get longer as the night progresses.

We all need more sleep time, and most of us would love to know how to sleep better. One in three of us is sleep-deprived, and that's dangerous to our careers, health, moods, and relationships. The first step is acknowledging the problem. Then, get more bright daylight in the morning and try one of the excellent sleep apps above. Chances are you'll soon be sleeping a lot better than a baby. Is sleep important?

Want to fall in love with sleep again? Here's how

Longevity; the art of graceful aging

We all know that a good night's sleep is a key ingredient for our health and wellness. There's science to back this up. Our bodies and minds need sleep—more specifically, REM (our deepest sleep)—to recharge and rejuvenate, down to the molecular level.

But, for many of us, sleeping has become a chore to be slotted into our packed schedules, with falling and staying asleep turning out to be more work than rest. We used to adore crawling into bed for a juicy night's slumber, and now we've got bed dread, a.k.a. sleep procrastination.

So why are we falling out of love with sleep? And more importantly, what's stopping us from reclaiming this precious gift of self-care we can give ourselves and our bodies? According to our informal survey of friends and family, the reason is life. Stress, work, technology, and over-programming our days all contribute to us getting less than the optimal amount of sleep. We know we're not doing ourselves a favor, but why can't we stop?

What are the signs of bed dread?

While you might spend all day looking forward to winding down and hitting the hay when the time comes, instead of turning off, your imaginary switch flicks to 'on'. You might go down any number of sleep procrastination rabbit holes, such as:

- Finishing just one or more household tasks

- Completing that last piece of work or checking emails one more time

- Getting caught up binge-watching a new 'it' show

- Convincing yourself to read just one more chapter

- Scrolling mindlessly through social media

Before you know it, it's 2 a.m., your ability to fall asleep easily has been tampered with and your sleep window has dramatically shortened.

So what can you do to turn life off so you can turn it in?

The good news is that sleep procrastination is not a permanent condition. You can fall in love with sleep again. The first step, like with anything else, is awareness of what's sabotaging your sleep. The next step is to take action.

Try implementing any or all of these easy fixes to two major sleep saboteurs and banish bed dread forever.

Stress: whirring mind, revved-up body that's what stress feels like. And when our minds are spinning, it becomes much harder to fall asleep. We know that life is full of stress, so the key is to find ways to manage how much it impacts our lives. Some strategies include:

- adding a physical outlet like regular movement to your day, even if it's a midday walk

- focusing on work/life balance and mentally leaving work when the proverbial laptop closes

- Downloading your to-do lists, worries, or thoughts—business and personal—into an agenda or journal.

- If you are working from home, set up your workspace away from your sleeping space so that you can separate those two parts of your life.

- engaging in a mindfulness and gratitude practice, including breath work and meditation

- Balancing stress with other enjoyable activities that 'fill your 'cup'—hobbies, sports, clubs, social time with friends and family

Sleep hygiene: Whether we want to admit it or not, we all thrive on routine, and one around bedtime is the key to quality sleep. Some ways you can improve your sleep hygiene are:

- Going to bed and waking up around the same time every day (yes, even on weekends!)

- being aware of how your body reacts to stimulants like caffeine and sugar and limiting those in the afternoons and evenings

- turning off technology—including TikTok—at least an hour before bedtime

- Setting reasonable boundaries for yourself around your TV time (no,

Netflix, we don't want to watch another episode)

- Create a calming wind-down bedtime routine for yourself, such as taking a warm bath or shower, reading a good book, listening to a podcast, or meditating.

- focusing on creating a restful sleep environment, such as incorporating soothing colors, soft lighting, or comfortable furnishings

- Making sure you have the right mattress and pillows for your sleep style

Your head hits the pillow, and even though you feel tired, you just cannot switch off. Your brain appears to be taking this very moment to contemplate life and the universe and to ask questions that can take you down a multitude of rabbit holes! For others, you fall asleep as soon as you get into bed, sleep for a few hours, and then wham! It is as if a light has been switched on; you are wide awake and unable to get back to sleep.

We all know how great we feel after a good night's sleep and the difference it makes in the day when we awake.

We can feel switched on, refreshed, full of energy, and raring to go. The day starts and ends positively. However, when we are struggling with our sleep, we can experience the exact opposite. We feel lethargic, unrested, and dreading the day ahead, as we know it is going to be a long, hard slog again!

Our cells go through a repair and rejuvenation process when we sleep well, and if we are not able to sleep, this regeneration is inhibited, and we see the effects of a lack of sleep on our physical well-being and also on our mental well-being. We can suffer from anxiety and the symptoms of depression, which can have a detrimental effect on our overall mental and physical health. We can be less motivated and less productive. As you can well imagine, this can have a real impact on our lives, not only our ones but our working lives too. It is in everyone's best interests to ensure they have a great night's sleep. So, what can we do to help us achieve this?

Managing the 'stress bucket'

This year has been a challenge for a lot of us. The changes involved in managing to work from home, juggling work life with homeschooling, and perhaps feeling isolated working from home rather than with a group of people have resulted in people's 'stress buckets' filling up and, for some, overflowing!

However, there are things that we can do that can help us deal with life, and these changes in a positive way will also help us to sleep better; in turn, when we sleep better, we will deal with life in a better way. Good eh? I have included a few tips below if you are one of those people struggling to sleep:

- Do your absolute best to go to bed at the same time and to wake up at the same time, even at the weekend or on your days off. The brain does respond well to routine!

- Talking of routine and how well the brain responds to it, it is best to make sure that your working day is structured in a way that is conducive to working well. So, make sure you start your day at your usual time, that you have a proper space to work from where possible, and that you have a proper lunch break away from your desk. Finish your day at the same time, as best you can. I can hear some of you saying, "But I don't have time for a lunch break!" Trust me on this one; you will be so much more productive when you take a lunch break. The brain does need to switch tasks or rest every 90 minutes, and when this happens, it boosts our energy levels!

- Make sure you plan your following day's tasks before you shut your laptop or PC down. You will start your workday knowing what you are aiming to achieve and will hit the ground running. The result is more productivity, which can make us feel good. And because we have planned the following day, we are not lying in bed thinking about it, which is keeping us awake!

- Practice thinking positively. I know this can be a hard thing to do when you are struggling with sleep, but we must train our brain to do this because then we activate the part of our brain that is much more sensible and intellectual and can deal with life in a much better way.

Thinking positively does not necessarily mean thinking about big things; it can be those small things too, like a conversation we have enjoyed or seeing the sun on a frosty winter's day.

- Make sure you come off any devices you may have been using during the evening about an hour before you go to bed, such as mobile phones, iPads, laptops, etc. Unfortunately, they omit an invisible blue light that affects the release of our sleep hormone, melatonin. The result is that the brain will find it difficult to switch off. It needs some time to 'come down' from the day. This is such an important aspect to consider. Why not take a nice relaxing bath or shower in that hour before you head off to bed, or listen to some nice relaxing music? Do not feel tempted to watch TV in bed either, as TVs omit the same blue light, which will have the same result on our brains! Bedrooms need to be a place of calm and rest.

- Check the room temperature in your bedroom; we tend to sleep better in a cooler room.

- Make time for you to relax. Practicing self-care is so important; it is not selfish; it is necessary. When we do this, we feel good, and when we feel good, everyone around us benefits, and we sleep well!

I hope you find these tips useful, and I wish you a wonderful night's sleep!

Chapter 6

The older you get the healthier you have been

Common conditions at an older age include hearing loss, cataracts and refractive errors, back and neck pain and osteoarthritis, chronic obstructive pulmonary disease, diabetes, depression, and dementia. As people age, they are more likely to experience several conditions at the same time.

People worldwide are living longer. Today, most people can expect to live into their sixties and beyond. Every country in the world is experiencing growth in both the size and proportion of older people in its population.

By 2030, 1 in 6 people in the world will be aged 60 years or older. At this time, the share of the population aged 60 years and over will increase from 1 billion in 2020 to 1.4 billion. By 2050, the world's population of people aged 60 years and older will double (2.1 billion). The number of people aged 80 years or older is expected to triple between 2020 and 2050 to reach 426 million.

While this shift in the distribution of a country's population towards older ages, known as population aging, started in high-income countries (for example, in Japan, 30% of the population is already over 60 years old), it is now low-- and middle-income countries that are experiencing the greatest change. By 2050, two-thirds of the world's population over 60 years old will live in low- and middle-income countries.

Ageing explained

At the biological level, aging results from the accumulation of a wide variety of molecular and cellular damage over time. This leads to a gradual decrease in physical and mental capacity, a growing risk of disease, and ultimately death. These changes are neither linear nor consistent, and they are only loosely associated with a person's age in years. The diversity seen in older people is not random. Beyond biological changes, aging is often associated with other life transitions such as retirement, relocation to more appropriate housing, and the death of friends and partners.

Older age is also characterized by the emergence of several complex health states commonly called geriatric syndromes. They are often the consequence of multiple underlying factors and include frailty, urinary incontinence, falls, delirium, and pressure ulcers.

Factors influencing healthy aging

A longer life brings with it opportunities, not only for older people and their families but also for societies as a whole. Additional years provide the chance to pursue new activities such as further education, a new career, or a long-neglected passion. Older people also contribute in many ways to their families and communities. Yet the extent of these opportunities and contributions depends heavily on one factor: health.

Evidence suggests that the proportion of life in good health has remained broadly constant, implying that the additional years are in poor health. If people can experience these extra years of life in good health and if they live in a supportive environment, their ability to do the things they value will be a little different from that of a younger person. If these added years are dominated by declines in physical and mental capacity, the implications for older people and society are more negative.

Although some of the variations in older people's health are genetic, most are due to people's physical and social environments, including their homes, neighborhoods, and communities, as well as their characteristics, such as their sex, ethnicity, or socioeconomic status. The environments that people live in as children or even as developing fetuses, combined with their characteristics, have long-term effects on how they age.

Physical and social environments can affect health directly or through barriers or incentives that affect opportunities, decisions, and health behavior. Maintaining healthy behaviors throughout life, particularly eating a balanced diet, engaging in regular physical activity, and refraining from tobacco use, all contribute to reducing the risk of non-communicable diseases, improving physical and mental capacity, and delaying care dependency.

Supportive physical and social environments also enable people to do what is important to them, despite losses in capacity. The availability of safe and accessible public buildings and transport, and places that are easy to walk around, are examples of supportive environments. In developing a public health response to aging, it is important to consider not just individual and environmental approaches that ameliorate the losses associated with older age but also those that may reinforce recovery, adaptation, and psychosocial growth.

What Do We Know About Healthy Ageing?

Stay Connected

Sign up for Healthy Ageing Highlights to get weekly emails about healthy eating, exercise, cognitive health, and more.

Many factors influence healthy aging. Some of these, such as genetics, are not in our control. Others—like exercise, a healthy diet, going to the doctor regularly, and taking care of our mental health—are within our reach. Research supported by the NIA and others has identified actions you can take to help manage your health, live as independently as possible, and maintain your quality of life as you age. Read on to learn more about the research and the steps you can take to promote healthy aging.

Taking care of your physical health

While scientists continue to actively research how to slow or prevent age-related declines in physical health, they've already discovered multiple ways to improve the chances of maintaining optimal health later in life. Taking care of your physical health involves staying active, making healthy food choices, getting enough sleep, limiting your alcohol intake, and proactively managing your health care. Small changes in each of these areas can go a long way toward supporting healthy aging.

Get moving: exercise and physical activity

Whether you love it or hate it, physical activity is a cornerstone of healthy aging.

Scientific evidence suggests that people who exercise regularly not only live longer but may also live better, meaning they enjoy more years of life without pain or disability.

Adults 40 and older found that taking 8,000 steps or more per day, compared to only taking 4,000 steps, was associated with a 51% lower risk of death from all causes. You can increase the number of steps you take each day by doing activities that keep your body moving, such as gardening, walking the dog, and taking the stairs instead of the elevator.

Although it has many other benefits, exercise is an essential tool for maintaining a healthy weight. Adults with obesity have an increased risk of death, disability, and many diseases, such as type 2 diabetes and high blood pressure. However, being thinner is not always healthier either. Being or becoming too thin as an older adult can weaken your immune system, increase the risk of bone fracture, and, in some cases, may be a symptom of the disease. Both obesity and underweight conditions can lead to a loss of muscle mass, which may cause a person to feel weak and easily worn out.

As people age, muscle function often declines. Older adults may not have the energy to do everyday activities and can lose their independence. However, exercise can help older adults maintain muscle mass as they age. In addition to helping older adults live better, maintaining muscle mass can help them live longer. In adults older than 55, muscle mass was a better predictor of longevity than weight or body mass index (BMI).

What can you do?

Although many studies focus on the effects of physical activity on weight and BMI, research has found that even if you're not losing weight, exercise can still help you live longer and better. There are many ways to get started. Try being physically active in short spurts throughout the day or setting aside specific times each week to exercise. Many activities, such as brisk walking or yoga, are free or low-cost and do not require special equipment. As you become more active, you will start feeling energized and refreshed after exercising instead of exhausted. The key is to find ways to get motivated and get moving.

Healthy eating: Make smart food choices.

Making smart food choices can help protect you from certain health problems as you age and may even help improve brain function. As with exercise, eating well is not just about your weight. With so many different diets out there, choosing what to eat can be confusing. Much of the research shows that the Mediterranean-style eating pattern, which includes fresh produce, whole grains, and healthy fats but less dairy and more fish than a traditional American diet, may have a positive impact on health. A low-salt diet called Dietary Approaches to Stop Hypertension (DASH) has also been shown to deliver significant health benefits. Lowers blood pressure, helps people lose weight, and reduces the risk of type 2 diabetes and heart disease.

Yet another eating pattern that may support healthy aging is the MIND diet, which combines a Mediterranean-style eating pattern with DASH. Researchers have found that people who closely follow the MIND diet have better overall cognition—the ability to think, learn, and remember—compared to those with other eating styles.

What can you do?

Try starting with small changes by adopting one or two aspects of the Mediterranean-style eating pattern, or MIND diet. Several studies have shown that incorporating even a part of these eating patterns, such as more fish or more leafy greens, into your daily eating habits can improve health outcomes. One study of 182 older adults with frequent migraines found that a diet lower in vegetable oil and higher in fatty fish could reduce migraine headaches. Another study that followed almost 1,000 older adults over five years found that consumption of green leafy vegetables was significantly associated with slower cognitive decline.

Even if you haven't thought much about healthy eating until recently, changing your diet now can still improve your well-being as an older adult. If you are concerned about what you eat, talk with your doctor about ways you can make better food choices.

Learn more about healthy eating and aging.

Getting a good night's sleep

Getting enough sleep helps you stay healthy and alert. Even though older adults need the same seven to nine hours of sleep as all adults, they often don't get enough. Feeling sick or being in pain can make it harder to sleep, and some medicines can keep you awake. Not getting enough quality sleep can make a person irritable, depressed, forgetful, and more likely to have falls or other accidents.

Sleep quality matters for memory and mood. In adults older than 65, researchers found that those who had poor sleep quality had a harder time problem-solving and concentrating than those who got good quality sleep. Another study, which looked at data from nearly 8,000 people, showed that those in their 50s and 60s who got six hours of sleep or less a night were at a higher risk of developing dementia later in life. This may be because inadequate sleep is associated with the buildup of beta-amyloid, a protein involved in

Alzheimer's disease. Poor sleep may also worsen depression symptoms in older adults. Emerging evidence suggests that older adults who were diagnosed with depression in the past and do not get quality sleep may be more likely to experience their depression symptoms again.

More generally, a 2021 study found that older adults who did not sleep well and napped often were at greater risk of dying within the next five years. Conversely, getting good sleep is associated with lower rates of insulin resistance, heart disease, and obesity. Sleep can also improve your creativity, decision-making skills, and even your blood sugar levels.

What can you do?

There are many things you can do to help you sleep better, such as following a regular sleep schedule. Try to fall asleep and get up at the same time each day. Avoid napping late in the day, as this may keep you awake at night. Exercise can help you sleep better, too, if it isn't too close to bedtime. Research suggests that behavioral interventions, such as mindfulness meditation, can also improve sleep quality.

Quit smoking

It doesn't matter how old you are or how long you've been smoking; research confirms that even if you're 60 or older and have been smoking for decades, quitting will improve your health. Quitting smoking at any age will:

- Lower your risk of cancer, heart attack, stroke, and lung disease.

- Improve your blood circulation.

- Improve your sense of taste and smell.

- Increase your ability to exercise.

Among men 55 to 74 years old and women 60 to 74 years old, current smokers were three times more likely to die within the six-year follow-up period than those who had never smoked.

What can you do?

If you smoke, quit. Quitting smoking is good for your health and may add years to your life. Nearly 200,000 people demonstrated that older adults who quit smoking between the ages of 45 and 54 lived about six years longer compared to those who continued to smoke. Adults who quit between the ages of 55 and 64 lived about four years longer. It is never too late to stop smoking and reap the benefits of breathing easier, having more energy, saving money, and improving your health.

Alcohol and other substances

Like all adults, older adults should avoid or limit alcohol consumption. Aging can lead to social and physical changes that make older adults more susceptible to alcohol misuse and abuse and more vulnerable to the consequences of alcohol. Alcohol dependence or heavy drinking affects every organ in the body, including the brain.

In addition to being cautious with alcohol, older adults and their careers should be aware of other substances that can be misused or abused. Because older adults are commonly prescribed opioids for pain and benzodiazepines for anxiety or trouble sleeping, they may be at risk for misuse and dependence on these substances. For adults aged 50 and older, misuse of prescription opioids or benzodiazepines is associated with thoughts of suicide.

What can you do?

Learn about the current U.S. guidelines for drinking and when to avoid alcohol altogether. It's important to be aware of how much you are drinking and the harm that drinking can cause. If you or a loved one needs help with substance abuse or alcohol use, talk with your doctor or a mental health professional. You can also try finding a support group for older adults with substance or alcohol abuse issues.

Go to the doctor regularly.

Going to the doctor for regular health screenings is essential for healthy aging. Getting regular check-ups helps doctors catch chronic diseases early and can help patients reduce risk factors for disease, such as high blood pressure and cholesterol levels. People who went to the doctor regularly also reported improved quality of life and feelings of wellness.

In recent years, scientists have developed and improved upon laboratory, imaging, and similar biological tests that help uncover and monitor signs of age-related disease. Harmful changes in the cells and molecules of your body may occur years before you start to experience any symptoms of the disease. Tests that detect these changes can help medical professionals diagnose and treat disease early, improving health outcomes.

What can you do?

Visit the doctor at least once a year, and possibly more depending on your health. You cannot reap the benefits of medical advancements without regular trips to the doctor for physical exams and other tests. Regular screenings can uncover diseases and conditions you may not yet be aware of, such as diabetes, cancer, and cardiovascular disease. If you only seek medical attention when you're experiencing symptoms, you may lose the chance of having your doctor catch a disease in its earliest stages, when it would be most treatable. Regular check-ups can help ensure you can start treatment months or years earlier than would have been possible otherwise.

Taking care of your mental health

Mental health, or mental wellness, is essential to your overall health and quality of life. It affects how we think, feel, act, make choices, and relate to others. Managing social isolation, loneliness, stress, depression, and mood through medical and self-care is key to healthy aging.

Social isolation and loneliness

As people age, changes such as hearing and vision loss, memory loss, disability, trouble getting around, and the loss of family and friends can make it difficult to maintain social connections. This makes older adults more likely to be socially isolated or to feel lonely. Although they sound similar, social isolation and loneliness are different. Loneliness is the distressing feeling of being alone or separated, while social isolation is the lack of social contacts and having few people to interact with regularly.

Older adults who are socially isolated or feel lonely are at higher risk for heart disease, depression, and cognitive decline. A 2021 study of more than 11,000 adults older than age 70 found that loneliness was associated with a greater risk of heart disease. Another recent study found that socially isolated older adults experienced more chronic lung conditions and depressive symptoms compared to older adults with social support.

Feeling lonely can also impact memory. A study of more than 8,000 adults older than 65 found that loneliness was linked to faster cognitive decline.

Research also shows that being socially active can benefit older adults. A study of more than 3,000 older adults found that making new social contacts was associated with improved self-reported physical and psychological well-being. Being social may

also help you reach your exercise goals.
A 2019 study found that older adults who had regular contact with friends and family were more physically active than those who did not.

What can you do?

Staying connected with others may help boost your mood and improve your overall well-being. Stay in touch with family and friends in person or over the phone. Scheduling time each day to connect with others can help you maintain connections. Meet new people by taking a class to learn something new or hone a skill you already have.

Stress

Stress is a natural part of life and comes in many forms. Sometimes stress arises from difficult events or circumstances. Positive changes, like the birth of a grandchild or a promotion, can cause stress too. Research shows that constant stress can change the brain, affect memory, and increase the risk of developing Alzheimer's or related dementias.

Older adults are at particular risk for stress and stress-related problems. How levels of the stress hormone cortisol change over time. Researchers have found that cortisol levels in a person's body increase steadily after middle age and that this age-related increase in stress may drive changes in the brain. Supports the notion that stress and anxiety rewire the brain in ways that can impact memory, decision-making, and mood.

Finding ways to lower stress and increase emotional stability may support healthy aging. In an analysis of data from the Baltimore Longitudinal Study of Ageing, scientists followed 2,000 participants for more than five decades, monitoring their mood and health. The data reveal that emotionally stable individuals lived on average three years longer than those who tended to be in a negative or anxious emotional state. Long-term stress may also contribute to or worsen a range of health problems, including digestive disorders, headaches, and sleep disorders.

What can you do?

You can help manage stress with meditation techniques, physical activity,
and participating in activities you enjoy. Keeping a journal may also help you identify and challenge negative and unhelpful thoughts. Reach out to friends and family who can help you cope positively.

Depression and overall mood

Although depression is common in older adults, it can be difficult to recognize. For some older adults with depression, sadness is not their main symptom. Instead, they might feel numb or uninterested in activities and may not be as willing to talk about their feelings. Depression not only affects mental health but also physical health. Although different from depression, which is a serious medical disorder, mood changes can also influence aging. A 2020 longitudinal study demonstrated a link between positive mood and better cognitive control. Further studies are necessary to determine whether changes that improve mood could improve cognition. The way you think about aging can also make a difference. Research shows that whether you hold negative or positive views about aging may impact your health as you age. Negative beliefs about aging may increase undesirable health outcomes, Alzheimer's disease biomarkers, and cellular aging. Meanwhile, positive beliefs about aging may decrease the risk of developing dementia and obesity.

What can you do?

Depression, even when severe, can be treated. As soon as you begin noticing signs, it's important to get evaluated by a healthcare professional. In addition to deep sadness or numbness, lack of sleep and loss of appetite are also common symptoms of depression in older adults. If you think you or a loved one may have depression, start by making an appointment to see your doctor or healthcare provider.

Leisure activities and hobbies

Your favorite activities are not only fun; they may also be good for your health. Research shows that people who participate in hobbies and social and leisure activities may be at lower risk for some health problems. For example, one study found that participation in a community choir program for older adults reduced loneliness and increased interest in life. Another study showed that older adults who spent at least an hour reading or engaged in other hobbies had a decreased risk of dementia compared to those who spent less than 30 minutes a day on hobbies.

Music, theatre, dance, creative writing, and other participatory arts show promise for improving older adults' quality of life and well-being, from better cognitive function, memory, and self-esteem to reduced stress and increased social interaction. Even hobbies as simple as taking care of a pet can improve your health. According to a 2020 study, pet ownership (or regular contact with pets) was associated with better cognitive function and, in some cases, better physical function.

What can you do?

Look for opportunities to participate in activities. Get out and about by going to a sporting event, trying a new restaurant, or visiting a museum. Learn how to cook or play a musical instrument. Consider volunteering at a school, library, or hospital to become more active in your community.

Taking care of your cognitive health

Cognition—the ability to think, learn, and remember—often changes as we age. Although some people develop Alzheimer's or other types of dementia, many older adults experience more modest changes in memory and thinking. Research shows that healthy eating, staying active, and learning new skills may help keep older adults cognitively healthy.

How different factors affect cognitive health

If you think your daily choices don't make a difference,

- At least 150 minutes per week of moderate- to vigorous-intensity physical activity

- Not smoking

- Not drinking heavily

- A high-quality, Mediterranean-style diet

- Engagement in mentally stimulating activities, such as reading, writing letters, and playing games

The findings show that making these small, daily changes can add up to significant health benefits. Those who followed at least four of these healthy lifestyle behaviors had a 60% lower risk of developing Alzheimer's. Even practicing just two or three activities lowered the risk by 37%. While results from observational studies such as this one cannot prove cause and effect, they point to how a combination of modifiable behaviors may mitigate Alzheimer's risk and identify promising avenues to be tested in clinical trials.

How cognitive training affects health outcomes

Many brain training programs are marketed to the public to improve cognition. Although some of these computer- or smartphone-based interventions show promise, there is some evidence that exercising your brain by learning a new skill can improve memory function. Adults 60 and older showed that sustained engagement in cognitively demanding, novel activities enhanced memory function. In particular, the new skills learned in this study were: 1) learning how to use computer software to edit photos, and 2) learning how to quilt. Learning a new game, instrument, craft, or other skill can be fun and may have the added benefit of staving off memory loss as you age.

Next step

Taking care of your physical, mental, and cognitive health is important for healthy aging. Even making small changes in your daily life can help you live longer and better. In general, you can support your physical health by staying active, eating and sleeping well, and going to the doctor regularly. Take care of your mental health by interacting with family and friends, trying to stay positive, and participating in activities you enjoy. Taking steps to achieve better physical and mental health may reduce your risk for Alzheimer's and related dementias as you age.

Chapter 7
Nutrition Biochemistry

The impact of nutrition on both physical and mental health has gained much interest in recent years. Emerging studies are finding stronger connections between diet, gut health, the microbiome, and various diseases (both physical and mental). Part of the research into these connections is being undertaken by the field of nutritional biochemistry, which investigates the mechanisms that underlie these interactions between diet and disease.

The biochemistry of nutrition recruits a multitude of scientific disciplines, including biology, chemistry, and physics, to gain a deeper understanding of aspects such as cell function and metabolism, clinical nutrition, macronutrients and energy, nutritional genomics, and other factors that contribute to the interplay between diet and disease.

What is good nutrition?

You've likely heard about healthy eating and nutrition since you were young. But what exactly does good nutrition mean? Nutrition is something that not only encompasses what you eat but also the nutrients and vitamins essential for you to thrive and stay on top of your health.

Longevity; the art of graceful aging

Food is an essential part of a good nutrition plan. Eating a variety of whole foods is the key to maintaining a healthy weight and body. But what else does a proper diet entail? According to the Centers for Disease Control, a healthy diet includes:

- Staying within your daily calorie intake

- Plenty of fruits and vegetables

- Emphasizing whole grains over processed

- Plenty of healthy proteins

- Nuts and legumes

- Meals low in saturated fats and trans fats

- Meals low in added sugars and cholesterol

It's easy to get caught up in eating processed foods such as chips and sweets, but they can wreak havoc on your overall health and weight. Moderation is the key to good nutrition. Making sure your daily food intake is healthy and made up of whole foods can help you reduce your risk of medical issues and help you age more gracefully.

What is the relationship between nutrition and aging?

Is there a link between your nutrition and aging? The truth is, that your nutritional needs change as you get older. As your body ages, it becomes more susceptible to certain conditions, which can be aggravated by a poor diet. Changes in your body also mean that you have different nutritional needs as you age.

Nutrition is always essential to your health, especially as you get older. Although eating well isn't always easy, it helps you keep your body in good shape and may help you prevent certain medical conditions in the future.

So how exactly you're dietary do needs change when you get older? There are a few physical changes that tend to affect your overall dietary needs, including:

- A slower metabolism

- Decreased bone density

- A smaller appetite

- Decreased lean body mass

- Trouble absorbing vitamin B12

All of these factors can make it difficult for you to get the right amount of calories and nutrients that your body needs as you get older. That means a lot of changes in your nutrition and diet, some of which include:

- Fewer calories are needed daily.

- Foods rich in vitamin B12

- Higher-quality protein foods

- Foods rich in calcium and vitamin D

- Understanding the need to increase your intake of food

It can be difficult to understand these changes until you're at the age where your nutritional needs change. However, our team of experts can help you prepare your body and eating habits gradually as you age. That puts you in a better position to maintain a healthy diet through the years.

How you can improve your nutrition

Improving your nutrition isn't something that happens magically overnight. When you've not been eating well for a while, it can take time to adjust. The first step to improving your nutrition is realizing that you have some work to do.

Eating a variety of foods is the best way to improve your nutrition. Each type of food has different vitamins and nutrients that each system in your body needs to function properly. That means you need fruits, vegetables, and lean proteins to sustain a healthy life.

Staying hydrated with water is another way to improve your overall health and nutrition. Hydration is also essential to many of your bodily functions, especially as you get older.

Nutrition as We Age

Good nutrition across the lifespan helps prevent chronic disease, and we know that it's never too late to make improvements to support healthy aging. Older adults are at greater risk of chronic diseases, such as heart disease and cancer, as well as health conditions related to changes in muscle and bone mass, such as osteoporosis. The good news is that this population can mitigate some of these risks by eating nutrient-dense foods and maintaining an active lifestyle.

Older adults generally have lower calorie needs but similar or even increased nutrient needs compared to younger adults. This is often due to less physical activity, changes in metabolism, or age-related loss of bone and muscle mass.

Preclinical studies provide ample evidence that several components of the diet, such as protein, carbohydrate, and fat content, as well as the intake of calories, play important roles in regulating aging processes, longevity, and the development of age-associated diseases, including cardiovascular and cerebrovascular diseases.

Special Considerations for Older Adults

The Healthy Eating Index (HEI) measures diet quality based on the Dietary Guidelines for Americans. Compared to other age ranges, older adults have the highest diet quality, with an HEI score of 63 out of 100.

Although this is very encouraging, there's still a lot of room for improvement. Eating more fruits, vegetables, whole grains, and dairy improves diet quality, as does cutting down on added sugars, saturated fat, and sodium. Support from health professionals, friends, and family can help older adults meet food groups and nutrient recommendations.

Eating enough protein helps prevent the loss of lean muscle mass. But older adults often eat too little protein, especially adults ages 71 and older. Since older adults are meeting recommendations for meats, poultry, and eggs, it's important to remind them that seafood, dairy-fortified soy alternatives, beans, peas, and lentils are great sources of protein. These protein sources also provide additional nutrients, such as calcium, vitamin D, vitamin B12, and fiber.

The ability to absorb vitamin B12 can decrease with age and with the use of certain medicines. Health professionals can help older individuals get enough vitamin B12 by ensuring that they're consuming enough foods, such as breakfast cereals. Older adults should talk with their healthcare provider about the use of dietary supplements to increase vitamin B12 intake.

Healthy Beverage Choices for Older Adults

Sometimes it's hard for older adults to drink enough fluids to stay hydrated because the sensation of thirst declines with age. Drinking enough water is a great way to prevent dehydration and help with digestion, and water doesn't add any calories! Unsweetened fruit juices and low-fat or fat-free milk or fortified soy beverages can also help meet fluid and nutrient needs. Healthcare providers can remind older patients to enjoy beverages with meals and throughout the day.

If older adults choose to drink alcohol, they should only drink in moderation—2 drinks or less in a day for men and 1 drink or less in a day for women. Remember that this population may feel the effects of alcohol more quickly than they did when they were younger, which could increase the risk of falls and other accidents.

Supporting Older Adults in Healthy Eating

Similar to other life stages, health professionals, family, and friends can support older adults in achieving a healthy dietary pattern that fits with their budget, preferences, and traditions. Additional factors to consider when supporting healthy eating for older adults include:

- **Enjoyment of food:** Sharing meals with friends and family can increase food enjoyment and provide a great opportunity to share a lifetime of stories, all while improving dietary patterns.

- **Ability to chew or swallow foods:** Experimenting with different ways of cooking foods from all food groups can help identify textures that are acceptable, appealing, and enjoyable for older adults, especially those who have difficulties chewing or swallowing. Good dental health is also critical to the ability to chew foods.

- **Food safety:** Practicing safe food handling is especially important for this age group. The risk of foodborne illness increases with age due to a decline in immune system function. Find more information on food safety for older adults and food safety for people with decreased immune system function.

What role can nutrition play in retarding aging?

In general, appropriate nutrition is crucial for aging since it can enhance the body's general health and functioning, delay the physical and cognitive decline that comes with aging, and lower the risk of contracting chronic diseases.

Additionally, healthy eating can enhance older adults' quality of life.

The bottom line

Longevity may seem beyond your control, but many healthy habits may lead you to a ripe, old age.

These include drinking coffee or tea, exercising, getting enough sleep, and limiting your alcohol intake. Taken together, these habits can boost your health and put you on the path to a long life. Breaking old habits and forming new ones is not an easy process, especially when it comes to foods you've been eating for your whole life.

Our diets are complex systems influenced by biological, cognitive, and social influences.

Therefore, a variety of tools may be needed to navigate those factors and stick to a healthy diet in the long term.

Nutrition is an essential part of health, and people can start leading a healthy lifestyle by making small changes to their diet.

It is also important to remember other key aspects of health, such as exercise and activity, stress strategies, and adequate sleep.